# YOGA

Importance of Anatomy Education for Yoga
Teachers

(Yoga for Weight Loss an Easy Beginners Yoga
Guide for Weight Loss)

**Kathleen Germann**

Published by John Kembrey

**Kathleen Germann**

All Rights Reserved

*Yoga: Importance of Anatomy Education for Yoga Teachers*
*(Yoga for Weight Loss an Easy Beginners Yoga Guide for*
*Weight Loss)*

ISBN 978-1-77485-154-8

Legal & Disclaimer

The information contained in this book is not designed to replace or take the place of any form of medicine or professional medical advice. The information in this book has been provided for educational and entertainment purposes only.

The information contained in this book has been compiled from sources deemed reliable, and it is accurate to the best of the Author's knowledge; however, the Author cannot guarantee its accuracy and validity and cannot be held liable for any errors or omissions. Changes are periodically made to this book. You must consult your doctor or get professional medical advice before using any of the suggested remedies, techniques, or information in this book.

# Table of Contents

INTRODUCTION ..................................................... 1

CHAPTER 1: WHAT IS YOGA NIDRA ................................... 5

CHAPTER 2: MINDFULNESS ........................................... 10

CHAPTER 3: HOW WILL YOGA BENEFIT YOU? .................. 16

CHAPTER 4: MEDITATION BENEFITS ............................... 22

CHAPTER 5: YOGA POSE FOR COGNITIVE BENEFITS AND
PSYCHOLOGICAL HEALTH ............................................. 33

CHAPTER 6: BREATH OF LIFE ........................................ 55

CHAPTER 7: GUIDED MEDITATION TO BOOST POSITIVITY 76

CHAPTER 8: MANTRA MEDITATION ................................. 84

CHAPTER 9: RETREATS AND COMMUNITY ..................... 118

CHAPTER 10: DESIRE - FOOD - SEX ............................... 123

CHAPTER 11: YOGA MEDITATION TO REDUCE STRESS ... 136

CHAPTER 12: RELEASE NEGATIVE OR STAGNANT ENERGY
AND EMOTIONS ......................................................... 139

CHAPTER 13: BENEFITS OF MEDITATION ...................... 150

CHAPTER 14: THE HEALING EFFECTS OF SLEEP .............. 162

CHAPTER 15: BREATHING MEDITATION ........................ 174

CONCLUSION ............................................................. 181

# Table of Contents

# Introduction

Losing weight is very difficult, and it appears that everyone has a specific idea about the right way to do it. The thing to understand is "one same size does not fit everyone," and this notion is quite fit when it comes to weight loss. Some simple differences such as people's age, sex, body shape, underlying medical conditions, physical activity, genetics, previous associations with dieting, and even dietary habits can affect a person's desire to losing weight and even maintaining it.

If you search the words "weight loss" on the web, you will find countless options and strategies available for weight loss, but people still fail more frequently to achieve weight loss or not regain the weight. Why does this happen? Do you have any idea?

Unfortunately, fad diets, various trends, and pills usually give you only immediate effects for some specific time. They will lead you to eat some foods or to avoid some foods, which sometimes frustrate people. And research shows that conventional diets frequently lead to little self-evaluation, anxiety, and depression. These emotions also stimulate the option of unhealthy foods, and the cycle continues. Therefore people gain more weight after getting some short-term results.

Most of us have concentrated on the wrong options when it comes to dropping weight. We haven't focused on our mind, the most important aspect of our body. So, instead of looking inward, we criticize and judge the 'program' or diet.

In eating and maintaining our weight and life, it is important to understand the link between the mind and the body. Our hectic, jam-packed lives will weigh us down. In a new survey, 38 percent of adults reported eating or overeating to prevent discomfort in the last month, and nearly 50% of these adults reported this as new habits.

If you can relate to this feeling or actions, you're not alone. The good thing is that only you can take action that can help you either control or lose weight. One of them is a meditation for weight loss. Now comes a question, what is meditation?

Meditation is essentially the process of directing your mind to become more alert. During meditation, the total attention flows inward instead of engaging in the outside world. Meditation practice will create good energy in you.

Many forms of meditation exist. Some of them are based around the use of some words called mantras. Others depending on breathing or focusing the mind at the present moment. Both these approaches will help you understand yourself better and how your mind and body function.

The increased awareness makes meditation a valuable method to help and understand your life patterns, leading to weight loss. Scientists have investigated and found out that meditation practice allows us to relax, sleep better, and improve our health. They also researched how meditation can help us in losing weight.

In recent research, scientists assessed how meditation could impact weight loss and some habits frequently related to unhealthy eating. They observed that guided meditation could minimize the level of emotional and binge eating. Other findings have also found that using stress-reduction strategies such as meditation can positively affect the weight loss journey.

Weight loss is not an easy task, and strong determination is required. But if you are ready to proceed, you will have comprehensive information in this book to help you lose weight and improve your life. So what are you waiting for? Keep reading this book to find a life-changing secret.

# Chapter 1: What Is Yoga Nidra

Yoga Nidra, a variant of yoga, is focused on providing a heightened level of being content with regards to contentment that is linked to your mentality, your emotions, and the physical composition of your own exterior and is an offshoot of meditation as well. I know what you're thinking: what is the point of trying to explore yoga Nidra when meditation is supposedly much more effective, and there are plenty of other yoga nuances that are more worthwhile to explore as well? Well, for starters, yoga Nidra helps curb your intensified and strong negative emotions that are penetrating your body as well as the bounds of your mind and helps to restore your sense of clarity and can provide some other kinds of benefits that are worth acknowledging as well. What exactly are the significant benefits that can arise through studying yoga Nidra and practicing it more frequently? There's the fact that through practicing yoga Nidra, this will offer assistance in treating any level of insomnia that you may find yourself combatting as well as help to lower the level of anxiety that you might be feeling or lower the impacts that are brought on as a result of being diagnosed with PTSD. If you find yourself reliant on utilizing chemical supplements or are facing agony that is frequent and consistent and does not go away after a certain period of time, practicing yoga Nidra can also help to diminish the influence of any or all of these factors as well. Suppose you are someone who has issues with repeating behavioral tendencies that are not a reflection of a healthy way of living, or perhaps you make poor decisions in terms of what you tend to do habitually throughout your daily life and have cognitive processes that are not exactly the most positive ones to have. If you find yourself in any or all of these given circumstances, you will definitely find that yoga Nidra can help you make the proper changes that are necessary to get your life back on track.

For those who still believe that meditation and yoga Nidra are one and the same, here are some tips that you can pay attention to in order to differentiate the two. For starters, meditation involves a person who remains seated, and while the person who is meditating might be in a position where they feel secure overall, he or she is not in a position where they are sleeping as he or she is still present and involved in the moment. When you are being attentive, typically within meditation, this means that for the most part, you are paying close attention to the mantra as well as your overall breathing habits, however; Meditation also follows the model of being able to guide you as well. Thus, this indicates that just because this person is seated with their eyes closed does not suggest in any means that the person who is in the midst of meditating is enduring a deep slumber where he or she is completely aware of their surroundings and what is going on, to begin with. I'm referring of course to their current position with regards to their overall consciousness, which is a term used to call someone who is for example, wide awake, completely focused and with a solid understanding of what is going on around them, or in a state where he or she has drifted off completely and has been able to block out all of the surrounding background noise and does not know what is going on. There is also not one exclusive state of consciousness that a person enters while he or she is meditating as people who practice meditating tend to fluctuate between various states related to a person's overall consciousness level, yet meditating mostly places people into a state of consciousness that mirrors what people resemble when they are just beginning to emerge from a restful slumber state after sleeping through the duration of the night. However, that being said, mediation can also bring people into a state of consciousness that is unique to being in a state where a person is waking from drifting into a deep sleep during the night, which is a state that is known as transcendental consciousness and people who practice meditation can also enter other states of consciousness when they meditate as well.

# Chapter 2: Mindfulness

Mindfulness is a popular concept based on both Buddhism as well as other types of Eastern philosophy, which has been merged into modern Western psychology. It is based on a few different principles. The most fundamental principle of mindfulness is the practice of being present. Mindfulness emphasizes the importance of being fully emerged in whatever you are doing at any given moment. This means not allowing your mind to drift into the past or worry about the future. The practice of living in the present moment has tremendous value. It means realizing that the past is in the past. All that we have is the present. Therefore, if we focus on the task at hand, we can see things objectively, and we can tremendously improve our thought process, our actions, and how we communicate.

Another important aspect of mindfulness practice is this concept of not only being present but also to be present without attaching your emotions or any type of judgement, as if you were a witness to everything that is happening. You can practice this throughout the day. For example, if you are driving in the car and screaming at another car that cuts in front of you, causing you to have to abruptly hit the brakes; be the witness of this. Imagine that you are in the passenger seat witnessing the whole scenario play out before your eyes.

Shakespeare's famous words ring truer than ever, "All the world is a stage, and all the men and women merely players". This concept is rooted in Eastern philosophy and the idea that all the material world is an illusion. This illusion is called Maya. It is this perspective of the world that has the power to ease suffering because we can look at the world in a completely different way. Suffering and misfortune can become part of a necessary process for growth or ascendance with the goal of transcending the obstacles that come our way. Imagine how powerful we can be when we simply continue to do what we are doing without overly attaching our emotions or reacting with fear?

In this way, we can dance through life with grace and focus. We approach each experience as if it is our first experience, being fully present. This concept of a beginner's mind can be practiced throughout the day. When you wake up in the morning and you hear the birds chirping, imagine you are hearing it for the first time, even if you have heard it a billion times before. While you are eating oatmeal, no matter how many times you have eaten the oatmeal, imagine that you are experiencing the taste and the texture for the very first time. When you are making love to your partner, experience it as if it was happening through the eyes and mind of a virgin! If you suffer from trauma, practice experiencing the thing that triggers you without attaching any emotion or meaning to it. Think of it as a traumatic experience as a tiny spec of sand in an entire dessert or a tiny star in a far, away universe.

Another important aspect of mindfulness practice is that it is effortless. You are not overly consumed with getting somewhere or attaining something. You are just being fully present with the task at hand. This does not mean that you cannot have goals, but it does mean that you want to avoid becoming overly attached to your goals to the point that you become emotional. This may lead to suffering.

If suffering arises, the key to easing the suffering is acceptance. Sit with your feelings without trying to suppress them. Resisting the experience will only prolong it. You must allow yourself to feel the feeling until it slowly dissipates. When you are reading a novel or watching a movie that brings emotion and makes you cry, eventually those feelings dissipate. In the same way, we must realize that suffering occurs but only time heals wounds. Of course, it is more difficult when the experience actually happened, but the key is transcending the ego and seeing things from the perspective that it did not just happen to the self. You move from the self to a witness of the self. It is an important part of the process of every human being to reach this kind of awareness.

Letting go is an integral part of a mindfulness practice. This means letting go of the past or the future so that we can receive the gift of the present moment. It means letting go of judgement and emotions, letting go of the fear of not attaining something, and accepting the moment for what it actually is, rather than what we think it should be or what we want it to be. The paradox is that when we let go, and we become fully immersed in the "now"...that is when the magic happens.

Mindfulness Meditation

Sit in a comfortable position. Look around the room. Notice the colors and the objects that are with you in the room. Examine each object in the room, one by one as if you were seeing it for the very first time, and without attaching any judgement to it. Be fully present. If you find your mind drifting into the future or into the past, pull it back to the present moment. Continue looking around and witnessing the sight in front of you as if you were a baby sitting on the lap of their mother or father. You have nowhere to go. You have nothing to do. Just sitting and looking around in awe of all the colors and all the shapes around you.

You can practice this short meditation when you are stressed, angry or overwhelmed with your feelings. It will allow you to come back into the present moment. It will allow you to return to the perspective of the silent witness.

# Chapter 3: How Will Yoga Benefit You?

Yoga, as a whole, can offer various benefits to your entire body. Just think about it: today we expose ourselves to various diseases, whether they be physical or mental. Yoga is very beneficial as it can help you not only clear your mind, but allow you to achieve what is truly important in life as well: good health and true happiness.

There are a variety of benefits to yoga and in this section we will explore those benefits.

1. Can Help Improve Mental Health

As many people are aware, with today's lifestyle it can be really hard to achieve optimum physical health and mental health at the same time. Yoga can certainly help with this. The core of yoga is about using proper breathing techniques along with proper postures to help enhance the health of your body. When you learn how to breathe properly, this allows the cells within your body to get the right amount of oxygen that they need for longer periods of time.

When you get the perfect amount of oxygen, your brain will benefit by improving your overall cognitive performance. By having more cognitive performance, you will have the ability to have more clear and concise thoughts that could improve your overall self-esteem and self-confidence.

2. Can Help Boost Your Overall Strength

Have you ever come home after a long day at work, crashed onto your sofa, and felt way too tired to even lift the remote for your TV? Many of us go through this on a daily basis and this is not something that occurs simply because we are tired. This occurs due to lack of inner strength.

There are various yoga poses available that can help enhance the strength within each and every one of us. Generating this inner strength is important to help us accomplish even the most basic of tasks on a daily basis and to avoid injuries that we can sustain from simply not paying attention.

### 3. Can Help Improve Your Flexibility

Many people today have the false pretense that in order to do yoga, you have to be flexible, when it fact it is actually the other way around. In order to become more flexible, you should do yoga. When you do yoga, it involves a lot of exercising and stretching throughout the entire process which has been shown to improve your overall flexibility while reducing the amount of pain that you feel.

### 4. Can Help Improve Cardiovascular Health

We all know how important our hearts really are. Without our hearts, we wouldn't be living. It's as simple as that. Developing a healthy heart system is necessary to prevent harmful and even fatal diseases, such as strokes, heart attacks, and high blood pressure. All of these diseases are caused by not only a poor family medical history, but by negative thinking, an improper lifestyle, and a poor diet.

5. Can Help Alleviate Sever Joint and Arthritis Pain

There are many people who suffer from inflammation and stiffness of their joints. When this happens, most people avoid exercising themselves. Yoga can help with this inflammation as it helps to prevent these kinds of ailments by helping to tone of the muscles within the body and by loosening the joints. When you use yoga, you have to go through a series of poses that will strengthen and stretch the muscles within your body. It also helps to enhance the blood flow going to the joints, muscles and tissues of your body that are stiff or sore. What does this mean? It means that your joints will be less painful and that you will be able to move more freely without any fear of pain.

6. Can Help To Prevent Respiratory Problems

There are many different yoga poses that, when done correctly, can act as a way to control a variety of respiratory problems, such as chronic asthma. How is this possible? When you practice yoga, it helps to increase the capacity and stamina of your lungs and eliminates the stress on the passageways of your lungs.

7. Can Help Improve Your Memory

Yoga, when used correctly, is meant to help you to focus on meditation and to improve your concentration. This can help you to hold in more information and to increase your memory for longer periods of time. There are various breathing techniques, meditating exercises, and concentration that you use when you do yoga. This can lead to an improved blood flow to your brain, which enhances the ability for you to accept and retain more information. If you are looking to stop suffering from short term memory loss, this is something that you should certainly try.

8. Can Help You Lose Weight

Losing weight is something that nearly all of us want to do. Obesity in many people today can be due to a variety of different reasons such as eating out of stress, hormonal imbalances, digestive imbalances, bad eating habits, and lack of exercise. By doing yoga, your body will take in even more energy, increase your metabolism, and break down fat cells. With the improved breathing that comes with doing yoga it helps to stimulate your abdominal organs to improve your digestion.

9. Can Help Combat the Effects of Ageing

Yoga helps to refresh both your mind and body and helps you to approach your life in a more positive and stress-free way. When you combine this new way of thinking with the flexibility, mental capacity, and enhanced fitness that yoga brings you, you will be practically glowing with new youth. If you want to feel and look younger, yoga is certainly one way to do it.

Now that you understand what the benefits of yoga are, the next thing for you to do is to begin practicing it. I will teach you how to do just that in the next few chapters so you can feel all these benefits for yourself.

# Chapter 4: Meditation Benefits

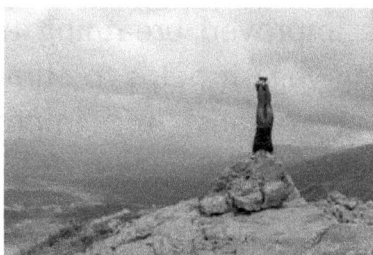

Meditation Benefits

Meditation will benefit you in relation to the effort you invest. The benefits can be far-reaching or elusive, and very often, both far-reaching and elusive. There is a cannon of scientific studies that have been undertaken that prove the positive influence that mediation has on the overall health of individuals who have taken up the practice. There are also the countless people that have engaged in it that have experienced first-hand the benefits of meditation and related their experiences to the wider world. It is a practice that has influenced religions from Buddhism and Christianity to esoteric spiritualisms the world over, and it has been adopted by some of the best minds of western science and arts, like Niels Bohr and Leonard Cohen.

It has been claimed that a steady dose of meditation can improve mood and psychological well-being, help treat a whole host of diseases, calm children suffering from ADHD, improve the chances of overcoming addictions, help you live longer, and make your life better in numerous ways. These are all really wonderful notions, but the most important thing that meditation will do for you, if practiced often, is the thing that you need it to do for you, whatever that may be.

It is said in the Buddhist tradition that you don't use meditation to become a better writer, or carpenter, or politician. You use meditation to become a better whatever-you-already-are. That is why I said the benefits of meditation can be elusive – you can never really tell what it is that will happen when you go down the rabbit hole, but you can bet it will matter in the context of your life and experiences.

It is difficult to write about the benefits of meditation because they are so subjective. When you undertake a tradition that is supposed to help you view yourself and reality in a clearer way it becomes almost ridiculous to try and communicate those experiences, like trying to communicate what it is like for you to see the color blue. But there are some almost tangible examples of what meditation can do for people when looked at in an empirical and scientific way. It actually works!

Take, for example, the work of Jeffery M. Schwartz and his treatment of patients with O.C.D with a treatment derived from his practice and adherence to mindfulness meditation, an aspect of Vipassana Buddhism. He theorizes that humans have the capacity to induce "self-directed brain plasticity," which is essentially the idea that the conscious directing of your attention can literally change the shape and biological functioning of your brain.

This theory is backed by extensive research and success with patients.

 People with O.C.D. experience intense and overwhelming fears that are only relieved when a compulsive activity is undertaken. This can be the fear of contamination and the compulsive desire to wash your hands over and over, or the fear that a loved one is going to die in the immediate future and the compulsion to open and close your bathroom door exactly twenty-three times is the only thing that can save them. These intrusive thoughts are very powerful versions of what Schwartz had experienced in his exploration of his own consciousness during meditation practice, which lead him to some insights.

He was convinced, much like the Buddha, that much of what directs our behavior and thoughts are hard-wired reactions to the world – we tend to be the puppets of our emotions and desires. The problem that O.C.D. patients have is that due to a biological functioning of the brain they have very intense and irrational emotions and desires. Since the practice of mindfulness is to view the thoughts and desires of experience with objective non-judgment, which would lead to a slow erosion of the power the thoughts and desires have over your consciousness, why couldn't that work with O.C.D patients as well?

Schwartz undertook to develop a program based on this mindfulness technique. He then instructed his patients on this technique and subjected them to brain scans which showed a remarkable change in the actual structure of the patient's brains. They had effectively rewired their brains to remove the faulty circuitry. It stands as one of the most convincing programs that empirically prove the effectiveness of meditation in improving the lives of people who practice it regularly.

The thing about these meditation-based secular practices it that they remove any tradition and ceremony from the practice which, for many people, add the depth and human touch. Many of the benefits of meditation center on the calming effects of the practice itself. But the studies that the secular practices are derived from are like a window into reality. They show that when meditation is undertaken the fight or flight centers of the brain are calmed. The subjective experience of this calmness is one of the most pleasurable and beneficial aspects of meditation, and one of the reasons people keep going back to the cushion.

Self-Control

Another benefit of meditation that has universal appeal is that it gives you a greater sense of self-control. When you begin to meditate it is essential that you first calm your mind and bring it to a place of stability and non-judgment. This will involve a great effort to focus your attention on to an image, a sensation, a mantra or any other object specific to your practice. When this is done it has the effect of putting you in a position to observe the intricate and personal workings of your mind. For so many people this is something that is sorely needed.

In many traditions, the mind is made up of various aspects that all work together to create a thing that you call you. These are feelings, thoughts, notions, ego and all manner of mental events that create the cyclone of activity that consistently flows through consciousness. You can identify with any number of these things that have their beginnings in any number of past events and future projections. By doing this you make up the story of you and use it to direct your behavior. One of the benefits of meditation is that it gives you the power to view this flow of mental activity from a point that you can more easily and effectively direct your attention to the aspects of your story that are beneficial to you, as opposed to becoming a slave to any thought or feeling that just happens to be the strongest one at that moment.

If you are visualizing you will be encouraged to focus on an image that you create in your mind and study the thoughts and emotions that come to the surface as you picture the mountain, lake, deity or whatever it is you are focusing on, instead of allowing the stream of mental events to carry you away.

If you are doing mindfulness meditation you will be encouraged to focus on your breath to the point that you have control over your attention. When you gain significant control over your attention through many hours of practice you can begin to position yourself in a manner that you will watch the flow of undisturbed thoughts and feelings as they pass through the eye of consciousness. In this way, you can study the way they relate to each other, the body, and the self.

These practices will cultivate an ability to sustain a greater sense of self-control throughout the day. It is a 'sense' of self-control in that, until you have learned to make decisions free of misplaced feelings or negative thinking patterns, you are still at the whim of the narrative you have tended to throughout your life, and you are basically falling into the same patterns that got you into needing to meditate in the first place.

Cultivating Compassion

Another great benefit of meditation is that it will foster compassion toward yourself and others. The need for compassion in our lives is great because it directs your behavior towards actions that will reduce the amount of suffering you and others will have to endure, and why else get into meditation other than to free yourself from suffering? Once you begin to see yourself as you truly are – not as a bad or flawed being but an ever-evolving consciousness – you will begin to understand that you are part of a greater whole and that actual freedom from suffering does not just involve you but all other beings as well.

The predominance of depression, mood disorders, general anxiety and panic, lack of good sleep, lack of sustained focus, and lack of good and wholesome sexual activity are all symptoms of a society that has turned against its true self. When big egos, self-satisfaction and attention seeking have become the goals of society there is little a person can do to fight the feeling of not being good enough or always wanting more. Cultivating a great compassion towards all the feelings and thoughts that bubble-up in your mind and attending to sense that you are already all you need be will help to bring the relationship to yourself to a healthy place.

It Will Help You Change Your Life

Gaining an understanding of yourself and the machinery of your mind can empower you to change your life in meaningful ways. There is a philosophy that informs most forms of meditation that come from India that lays out the universal workings of the machine. There are multiple aspects of your mind that all work together to create the thing you call yourself.

When you stabilize you mind with meditation it is possible to see how these aspects are all separate things that can be isolated and investigated. With this investigation will come the power to make choices that are not guided by misplaced or unfounded feelings or thoughts. With an understanding of what you are you can reshape your life. You can change your ways if you learn how to harness your mind.

# Chapter 5: Yoga Pose For Cognitive Benefits And Psychological Health

Practicing yoga can usually decrease pain, depression and anxiety and give the attitude and sense of well-being a big boost. But there are a few positions you can do to address this field directly, as well as improve your executive capacity and increase memory, intellectual comprehension and intellect. To these ends, Surya namaskara is excellent, as mentioned above.

And so. Better are backward-bending poses, such as camel pose, bow pose and spine twisting poses, such as waist-rotating pose and Ardha matsyendrasana or half-spinal twist, as mentioned in this segment. We can add upside-down poses that increase blood flow to the brain, such as vipareeta Karani asana (inverted pose) and its more comprehensive system, Sarvangasana (shoulder hold, not mentioned in this book).

3.1    Sitting Bend:

If Ardha matsyendranasana, or the half spinal twist, is a little too complicated for you, you can try this "sitting twist," which is easier and less difficult. Lie in a relaxed pose, in sukhasana. Twist around to the left. Place the left hand

Hand, palm down, your right-hand lies on your left hip, on the floor behind you. Without stretching, tilt your back as far as you can, and you look past you. Keep the position for twenty minutes, relaxing slowly and letting your back, chest, neck and shoulders fully relax. Return to sukhasana then repeat on the right.

Advantages: This posture is profoundly calming, reducing fear and tension. It gives the spine a slight twist from the base all the way to the shoulder, thus bringing strength to the back and strengthening posture.

3.2    Half Spinal Twist

From a sitting posture, with legs spread out before the body, bend Place your right foot flat on the floor and knee right. Move the left leg and put the knee under the right leg's crook, so that the left foot can hit the right butt cheek. Take the left arm to the right side of the body and the other hand of the right hip, and grab the left foot. The left-arm will be pushed against the right hip.

Hold the neck upright, exhale and flip the body to the right-hand-side and Place on the floor with your right hand, elbow closed. Twist your neck to the right so far as it is possible to apply to this pose's bent angle, but don't let your shoulders lean back. Hold your neck high and straight.

The concept is to use your right leg and left arm to twist the backbone without having to Use the muscles of the back, so the muscles of the spine and back are left to relax completely. In that Place, you shouldn't struggle or push something. Breathe intensely for twenty breath counts, then inhale and return gradually to starting spot. Redo then the entire position, this time on the left side.

Advantages: Half spinal twist helps to relieve stress, anxiety and depression. It does help Deep strain escape from the back, shoulders and arms, frequently followed by pain. This is also an effective backstretch that extends and strengthens the muscles on either side of the back in turn, which can strengthen back issues such as a slipped disk.

### 3.3    Half Inverted Pose

This posture is a rehearsal for the correct Karani vipareeta, in which you are Raise your legs straight up without assistance while allowing the weight of your arms.

Put a pillow, or two, next to a wall in this preparatory pose. Would you want to Place your butt and lower back on the mattress, while your legs point straight up to the wall? Their arms and hands are lying on the surface. Thus your chest and shoulders will be substantially higher than your hips. When you're in line, you should just relax and breathe deeply like that. Bring your knees to your chest to return from this asana, and then lift them onto your shoulders hand, before getting up.

Advantages: Half inverted pose overturns the normal gravity direction at the body. Blood flows from the legs and passes into the upper part of the body. The improved blood supply to the brain usually increases the thought and learning, as well as provides relief and stress reduction. If your work or way of living is not very productive and you are sitting for extended periods Time, the pose is of particular support. It should help to reduce any possible swelling or discomfort in the foot and legs. Overall it increases circulation.

Contraindications: Give this one a miss if you have elevated blood pressure, as it will raise blood pressure in the upper body.

3.4     Inverted Pose

Lie flat on the ground, together with your feet. You should have your arms at your side, hands against the board. Breathe in as you lay down. Then catch the breath, raise your legs to the ceiling and take them to your back. Pressing you're hands down, letting your shoulders do the job, and raising your hips off the concrete, which would allow your back to curve.

Push the hands up but leave the elbows on the surface, then put the hands just below the hips to stabilize the weight on the lower section of the body. When that's too rough, instead, you should keep your hands to your butt cheeks. Your knees and shoulders carry the body weight.

Keep your legs up to the floor at an angle of 90 degrees. Close your eyes and watch out Relax and relax naturally for as long as you are at peace.

Then hold in your breath, raise the knees up to your shoulders, face down your hands to the floor, and gradually lower the buttocks to the floor, eventually rest the legs and assume the original position. You may find it much easier to prop up your legs against the wall at first while also retaining this pose.

Advantages: Inverted position reverses the tidal force on the body, which has a variety of benefits. It particularly triggers an increase in blood pressure to the brain. The improved blood supply through the brain strengthens the mind, relieves fear, stress and depression, boosts executive skills, and enhances memory and intelligence. Inverted posture frequently relieves hemorrhoids and flatulence.

3.5     Serpent Pose

Lie on your hands lying on your back. Lace your hands underneath your back together, and put them on your butt cheeks. Place your head on the table. When you inhale, uplift your shoulders as far as you can from the surface. Start engaging the muscles of your rear for this, but do not push it. Lift your arms, at the same time. Look away.

Hold this posture without inhaling, for as long as you can. And gradually reduce your shoulders once more to the ground as you breathe out. Turn to one side of your head, and loosen up. Do some rounds.

Advantages: Apart from being an ideal way of reinforcing the lower spine, the serpent posture extends and lifts the arms. It soothes respiratory illnesses like asthma. Fostering air circulation and a healthy heart is beneficial. It also helps you to relinquish any negative feelings that you may hang onto.

3.6     Yoga Poses for Looking Younger

Typically speaking, any reversed poses will counteract the influence of inertia on your skin, making you look youthful and heading off the appearance of drooping facial characteristics that make you look old. Through this way, Surya namaskara and the reversed pose (above) through general are helpful. Another popular posture for keeping a youthful look is halasana, the plow posture.

Plough Pose

Lay flat on your back and your arms and legs to your backs, with the hands facing downwards. Breathe in and lift your legs without lowering them from the ground freeing your muscles to do the job. Hold your chest, and force your hands and arms to the ground to raise your butt and neck, vertebra by vertebra, in a circular gesture to your heart.

Drop the legs over your shoulders before the feet hit the ground behind your knees. When you can't get this far enough, don't push it.

You can either keep the position by pushing the hands to the surface or bend the elbows to move the hands to the rear so that they can assist you. Keep the position as long as you feel relaxed and take a deep breath, enabling the muscles to contract, especially in the neck and upper back.

The initial supine posture can be restored by gradually lowering the spine, vertebra by vertebra, to the ground, then the butt, then feet. When you've kept your hands to your thighs, bring them face down to the ground first, then lower spine, butt and feet.

Another way to get into the plough posture is to continue with the reversed pose (above) or its more developed variant, Sarvangasana, posture.

Advantages: Plough posture has many benefits, like encouraging a healthy glow by making blood circulate to the nose. This also improves the stomach muscles and massages the intestinal organs and facilitates digestive health. It extends and improves back and neck muscles, reducing strain from the neck and shoulders and growing blood supply to that area. Plough pose and upright pose will also raise acne.

Warrior Position I

The warrior posture series includes three poses, the third of which is quite stubborn. Such poses are ideal for toning the thighs, ass, neck, back, and shoulders muscles, as well as promoting movement and maintaining a youthful look. They also create a sense of youth confidence and bravery, keeping your vision more potent and more concentrated – a committed warrior's attitude.

This set of three poses is named after Virabhadra, a mythical hero. The first posture imitated his mentality when Shiva commanded him to rise from the ground with the blades in his hands penetrating the sky.

Stand by your sides with your weapons upright. Cross your body around your Face, palms touching. Extend your legs out when you inhale, so that they reach about two-thirds of your size. Then breathe out while turning to the left. Spin the left foot at the same time, so that it points in the same position. Buckle your left leg and turn in that position, with your back arched with your arms still pointed upward with your eyes moving around your head to your side. The right leg will be straight behind you and extended.

Keep the pose for five seconds, and then loosen the left leg once more. Rotate the left foot back to its point of roots. Turn right then, rotate the right foot, and repeat right side position. Continue on for 5 to 10 cycles. Then breathe out to get back to standing.

Advantages: Warrior stance, I strengthen chest, foot, back, shoulders, and arms muscles. This stretches the legs and thighs too. It's improving order. Warrior stance I improve focus as well.

Pose Warrior II

The second posture of the fighter imitates the attitude of Virabhadra when he saw his distant rival.

And again, spread the legs out to the same depth as before from the same standing posture. Extend the limbs parallel to the wall on either side. Then, twist the left foot again until it faces out to the left. Lean with your left leg in that position, and bend your knee. Hold right out. The eyes will travel down the left neck. Keep the pose to a five-count.

Then come back to flat, extended spot. Make the same right-hand motions. Redo for 5 to 10 cycles, and then move to the initial standing position.

Advantages: Warrior posture II strengthens the muscles of the thighs, their shoulders and back. It increases stability. This psychologically builds a sense of bravery.

Warrior Pose III

The third posture of the fighter imitates the stance of Virabhadra as he progresses, cutting his enemy's head off with his dagger. This one is complicated and appears like something from a Kung Fu movie. You should do the third Virabhadrasana until you're confident with the previous two poses of the warrior.

Continue standing upright again, and adopt the squared pose again with legs spread apart. Switch your left leg until it faces the back. Then, exhale; raise your right foot off the floor together with your whole body turning to the side, arms spread out all the way.

The goal is to create a kind of T-shape, with your whole weight Placed on the left leg, the right leg stretching out behind you and your arms spread out in front of you. And much of the body is parallel to the table. Keep the equilibrium for a five-count, if you may. When you can't hold it too long, go back to squared position — and try not to slip! (But if you do, there's no big deal. Just rinse and wash.) Wash again on the right.

Advantages: Virabhadrasana III improves strength and coordination. Even because it mimics an intensely concentrated sword attack, this asana increases attention and discipline. It conditions the leg muscles and supports the heart.

3.7    Yoga Poses for Relaxation

Our lives are so crazy and frenetic these days, especially at such a young age. We are so excited about the innovation that we stay active even when we get some time to relax, streaming into our heads a relentless stream of data. The consequence is that we never, if ever, take time to teach ourselves compassion by merely relaxing. Unfortunately, we may not even be able to relax.

Resting doesn't just mean resting or lying down, even though it may even mean that. Resting can also involve taking the opportunity to do yoga, or enjoying your favorite meal, or landscaping — if that's the kind of thing you find fun and calming. Ultimately, it can be called rest something you do for internal pleasure, and that makes you feel refreshed and healthy.

For any meditation activity relaxing is necessary. If you don't take your time to relax, you'll be sick in body and mind. The positions in this chapter are intended to bring about a condition of physical and mental relief.

Corpse Pose

Lay somewhat apart on your back with your knees, and rest your arms a few inches apart from each side of your torso, palms up and together. Close your eyes, and let both your body and mind relax. If you like, you should concentrate your attention on the air mentioned in the meditation section, enabling your focus to connect with the wind and interact with that. Through this way, the body and mind enter a state of intense and usual calm.

You should sit in the posture of a corpse as long as you want. This usually comes at the close of a yoga session, so if you are physically or emotionally exhausted and need to relax, you should also lie down in Shavasana. Time and repetition will improve your attention to your needs, so that when you need to relax. You are well-tuned.

Advantages: Corpse posture allows for full body and mind relief. It helps the muscle fibers to rebuild itself, which reduces pain and anxiety.

It lets you regain your strength, particularly after a rigorous session of practice. Heart pressure is rising, and compulsive overthinking is relaxed.

Reversed Corpse Pose

Lay back with your legs spread on your chest, the tips of your feet spread over the concrete. You should extend the arms out, with the palms pointing downwards. Place your head back on the floor. Enable all of your body's muscles to relax fully, and breathing naturally, without pushing or altering anything about breathing. As with corpse pose, here you may want to practice breath-awareness, counting from one to ten to promote deeper relaxation. Hold the Place for as long as you want, just relaxes without any worries.

Advantages: Similar to the corpse pose, an inverted corpse pose makes a deep relaxation of the body-mind system. It is also useful for slipping joint, neck pain, and for improving bad posture.

Crocodile Position

Lay flat on the back, like in inverted posture of the dead, aiming at the feet. From the floor, raise your head and chest and Place your hands in your hands to relax, protecting it with your elbows. Let your entire body and muscles relax. Shut your eyes; breathe normally, without having to change your breath.

If your neck has too much pressure, push your elbows apart for a gentle lowering of your shoulders. You should feel the same weight on your neck and lower back, so you should change your elbows to find the right balance. Without tension, the body should feel calm and happy. Hang posed in crocodile for as long as you want to.

Advantages: As with the posture of the deceased and the pose of the inverted body, crocodile pose causes a relaxation response and reduces stress and anxiety. It also enhances such spinal conditions as a slipped disc as an inverted corpse pose. Crocodile pose has one significant improvement over the preceding two postures: it makes it possible to breathe slowly from your abdomen, use the diaphragm rather than the lungs to take the oxygen.

Risk factors: Do not pose with a crocodile if it makes you feel some pain in the back.

Sphinx Position

Lay upon your stomach on the ground. Your toes will extend downward. Touching the ground with your palms and elbows, breathe in and drive with your back, lift your stomach, head and shoulders off the ground. Your navel will hit the floor regardless. Your head will be kept straight up, like the sphinx facing ahead—calming breaths and softly, keeping a countdown to ten at the spot. And again, gently lower yourself back to the board.

Advantages: Sphinx posture fortifies the neck. The belly and stomach muscles are extended, facilitating metabolism. The neck and shoulders extend. This posture promotes movement and reduces emotional tension.

Cow's Face Pose

Sit on the floor with your knees out and straight back, palms leaning on your thighs. Place your left foot behind your right leg, and put it on your right hip outside. Then lift your right foot off your left leg and place your right foot behind your left knee. Knees on top of each other would be one.

Breathing, stick out your left arm horizontally. Shift your palm down first, then upwards, so that your thumb faces downwards. Breathing deeply, put the arm across your back and put it to your bottom. And as far as possible, push the arm up the neck, holding it to the left of the backbone.

Breathe and straighten out the right arm. Open the hand up, and raise the neck upwards. Breathe it out, and fold it over your head and back. Seek to find the best side if you can. Hang on for one or two minutes. Then untwist your palms, go back and return to the initial spot, alternating right and left.

When the hands are unable to touch each other, using a brace, hang it off your shoulder, then snatch it with your bottom hand. This even catches the cord as the upper hand comes off the ear and stretches downwards. Then raise the lower one with the upper arm to extend. Don't worry-the the goal is to maximize versatility slowly.

Advantages: The facial posture of Cow covers the hands, shoulders, neck, back and arms. It lifts the shoulders and reduces back, neck and shoulder rigidity. It is an excellent therapeutic way to alleviate stress and discomfort. When you are sleepy, it recovers strength and strengthens your stance.

Staff Pose

Sit down with your knees out in front of you and flat on the concrete. Keep the rear straight and erect. Place your hands behind you, palms flat on the ground. That may be painful if the hamstring muscles are tight. In this case, try having the correct spot by sitting directly against a wall with your back.

Advantages: Staff pose enhances your core muscles, helps stabilize your spine and seated bones and encourages posture.

Reclining Twist

Sit as in Shavasana on your back, with your weapons at your feet. Bend your left leg and put your foot to the side of your right thigh. You were using your right hand to grab your left leg and lower it to level.

Extend the left arm to the left and allow it to sit on the concrete, palm up. Turn your face as far as you can towards the west, and look in that position. Do not raise your shoulder blades off the table. Keep on for a minute and calm. Switch than in the other direction.

Advantages: The reclining twist increases spinal strength. It boosts the internal cavity. This relaxes and broadens the thighs and arms. This eases the fear and tension. It enhances metabolism, as well.

Eagle Position (in sitting position)

Start in a sitting position. Bend your right leg behind your left thigh, and Place your foot behind your left hip. Then carry the right foot out of the left hip. The left leg will sit on the right-hand arm.

Then have your wings spread out before you. Hold your arms upright, a little over the knees; pass your right arm over your chest. Bend the left elbow while holding the right arm upright. Your left palm is to the right.

Then extend your right shoulder, turning your palm to the right. Push right-hand palm and left-hand fingertips. If that's not necessary, otherwise use the left hand to grip the right thumb. Lift your wrists in such a way that your upper arms are at the right angle. Additionally, your upper arms should be straight, so that your elbows form a right corner too. Keep the pose for the duration of 10 to 20 breaths, breathing heavily into the space between the blades of your shoulder.

Advantages: For easing muscle strain in hard-to-reach regions of the upper back and neck, this posture is second to none. You'll definitely notice it touching long-neglected muscles right away, which required some tender loving treatment. Raise your elbows slightly if you want to offer a little added stretch. There's a more technical, standing variant of this pose that needs excellent pull-out stability and concentration. But I introduced the simplified version here as an example, so you can automatically get the advantages of that role.

# Chapter 6: Breath Of Life

It has a practical purpose. Breath is an evolutionary force that forces us to enter into relative existence and manifests there until - also through breathing - we evolve to the readiness to return to the original state. To return from the diversity of relativity and return to our original unity, we must focus our understanding on the original impulse to the duality that is most objectively manifested. is a physical process by which we inhale and exhale. In fact, these two movements seem to be one, inseparable, and together have the potential to return us to our origins and ours. Thanks to our full attention to the whole process of inhaling and exhaling, we immerse ourselves in the more subtle levels of this alternating cycle, moving to deeper levels and deeper until we finally reach the starting point. Then, thanks to this double movement, we regain our lost unity. By constantly practicing this transcendence, we will establish ourselves in this unity and be free forever from all forms of bondage, the attainment of Nirvana: forever unbound. That is why the modern Thai master of Buddhism Ajaan Fuang Jotiko said: "Breath can take you to Nirvana" and Sri Ma Anandamayi, perhaps the most famous spiritual figure of India entering the second half of the twentieth century said: "Nothing can be achieved without cultivating the breath." This is done through a process that is simply called breathing meditation because breathing is both an entrance and an exit.

The Path to right Breathing

1) Sit upright, comfortable and relaxed, put your hands on your knees or hips, palms down or palms down or up, on the other hand, on your knees.

2) Slightly point your eyes down and gently close them. This removes visual distractions and lowers your brain actions by about 75%, thus helping to still your mind.

3) Your mouth should be closed so that all breathing is through the nose. It also contributes to the serenity of the mind. Even though you keep your mouth open,

the jaw muscles should be relaxed so that the upper and lower teeth do not contract and do not touch, but separate.

4) Inhale and exhale slowly and deeply three to four times, feeling the inhale and exhale move inward and outward through the nostrils.

5) Now breathe naturally and easily, keep your consciousness on the tip of your nose, feel the breath when it flows in and out of your nostrils. (Some people know more about the end of the nose or more than half an inch or more, others know more about the end of the nose, and others know more about the nostrils. What happens naturally is best for you. Whenever this book says "nose tip," this applies equally to these three areas.) Do not watch the inhale and inhale the body, just notice the sensation of breathing on the tip of the nose.

6) Keep your consciousness on the tip of your nose, breath naturally and calmly, easily observe the sensation of breathing moving there during inhalation and

exhalation. This makes it easy to enter the Witness Consciousness that you are.

7) Do this until the end of the meditation, let your consciousness gently lean on the breath on the tip of the nose and feel the sensation of breathing moving there. After a while, you may feel as if the breath and discharge from the tip of your nose exceed your actual nostrils, or you may not feel your nose at all, but just breathing moving in front of your nose lies. This is normal, but the focus of your attention should be only on this, not on one. But the focus of your attention should be only this point - and not somewhere else outside or inside the body.

8) Let the breath go as you like. If the sigh is natural, so be it. If it is short, leave it as is. If the inhale and exhale are not the same length, this is normal. Let the breathing be natural, not forced, but just watch and experience it.

Breathe awareness

We do not need to control our breathing, but only to feel it, because if we fix our awareness of it and allow it to move at will, it will lead us to an ideal mental consciousness. The perception of simple breathing actually frees the breath - and our consciousness - from the congestion and immobility that we create, which are not in harmony with the cosmic order, the main purpose of which is evolution through conscious development.

Breathing is the primary manifestation of duality, and at its core is the unity of pure perception. Breathing itself combines both energy and consciousness. When we look at its nature, we see that respiration is not a "thing", but a process that can draw us to the core from which it arises - may be conscious - to change on all our levels exist. Awareness of breathing generates awareness of awareness, mental awareness.

There are two breaths, the outer breath and the subtle inner breath that creates it. By focusing our awareness on external respiration, we allow ourselves to perceive internal respiration. Having reconciled with them, we are immersed in the spirit from which they come from their roots.

Observing the breath unleashes the spiritual-spiritual consciousness, including the spiritual will. In this way, the spirit controls and governs our lives.

We hold our consciousness both on the inhale and on the exhale, as they are a manifestation/reflection of the two poles found in all existing objects. The subtle currents emitted from these two poles became all forms of energy in the physical and subtle bodies. These currents stroll outward and are demonstrated as inhalation and exhalation. In the body, two breaths are the forces of yin and yang, yin and yang, which act on both sides of the meditator. In the end, they are one, and every breath brings us unity.

In all relative beings, the breath of prana has become damaged and confusing, which binds consciousness rather than frees it. It was not in phase, not in rhythm or not in key features - outside the original, natural pattern of movement. Deeply observing his breathing, the meditator rearranges and redraws it, easily restoring its original appearance and function. In this way, it enters directly into the growing stream of evolution and accelerates its movement in it.

Effectiveness of attention

The Buddha calls breathing meditation Anapanasati. Anapana means inhaling and exhaling. Sati means intentional attention, not just unintentional perception. At first, in practice, we are simply aware of breathing, but after a while, we will find that breathing makes us aware of the very attention. Then Anapanasati means awareness created - or inherent - in the breath.

You can pray, sing, or chant mantras without paying attention to them — even thinking about other things — but you cannot practice noticing breathing on the tip of your nose without knowing it. Awareness of breathing ensures that the yoga mind remains unambiguous. As the Gita says, "The light of a lamp does not flicker where there is no wind: it is an analogy of a one-end practitioner" (Bhagavad-gita 6:19).

Although we tend to think of attention as a state of mind, as opposed to inattention, it is actually a wonderful spiritual force. Quantum physics has found that when people pay attention to something, the object is instantly affected to some extent - to such an extent that the scientist can inadvertently influence the result of the experiment, although external conditions can be controlled. The thought is really a thing, but attention is the main force of thought.

When we calmly adjust our perception of breathing, it becomes thinner, gentler, and more pleasant, often as light as the breeze of a butterfly's wings. The finer the breath, the closer the awareness to the Ego, and therefore the easier and happier the experience. To fully experience the breath is to feel the Ego. When sighing disappears, self-awareness remains. Because it is natural for breathing to breathe cleaner and cleaner during viewing, there is no need to consciously do so. Your attention will automatically improve it. As we become more aware of the subtle forms or movements of internal breathing, it automatically happens that the movement of breathing at all levels becomes slower. For pranayama, this is the peak.

The more we pay attention to the breath, the thinner it becomes until it manifests as an act of the mind, including the mind itself (chitta). Breath, like an onion, has many layers. In the practice of breathing, breathing, we feel these layers, starting from the most objective, material levels and gradually moving to ever thinner layers, until, as with the onion at its base. , there are no more layers, but only pure being (consciousness). Breathing becomes purer as we observe it, and as a result our perception becomes purer.

When breathing seems restless, or uncomfortable, or somehow dissatisfied, the simple force of attention (sati) does everything right. It is important to realize that because when we are dissatisfied with such breathing, we are really dealing with congestion or confusion at various levels of ourselves. If we try to fix or send them out, we can make them worse. But calm and carefree observation/perception of breathing, ignoring its temporary qualities, will do everything right, eliminating these blockages or problems. This is especially true. So just keep watching - relaxed attention will take care of all this.

The tip of the nose as a reference point

In Hindu, Buddhist and Taoist traditions, meditators should pay attention to the tip of the nose. This is obviously of practical importance to provide us with a stable starting point so that our mind does not waver during meditation. But there is much more to this than the faithful meditator will discover. The tip of the nose is the best place to focus attention and the best for subtle perception. Awareness of Nosetip ensures that you do not get lost in the many threads or streams of a fine breath of prana, but will only perceive the streams of inhalation and exhalation (prana / apana), which are the center of respiration mental breathing.

In relative existence we are constantly caught between two poles, both empirically and philosophically: form and formlessness, duality and unity, incarnation and discreteness, connectedness and liberation, unconscious and conscious, material and spiritual, infinite and finite. Unfortunately, we tend to think about choices and identify with each other when we need to overcome them. During breath meditation, we focus our attention on the tip of the nose, because it is neither inside nor outside the body and therefore the point of attention we can slide rather than touch and beyond the poles that connect us.

The Buddha never left the tip of his nose in his meditation instructions, and classical Buddhist meditation manuals and modern Buddhist teachers are quoted in the chapter on traditional Buddhism of this book. The Buddha taught that when we begin to breathe, we must pay attention to the parimuha, which means both "in front" and "in the mouth" - in other words: the tip of the nose. It should be understood that the "tip of the nose" means more than the cartilage and skin of the nose, which is the point at which the subtleties of our existence correspond to the physical tip. This is where the real breath is felt.

Since this form of meditation is called breathing meditation, we must not forget that our relaxed awareness should always be higher / breathing. To do this, we observe our breathing at the tip of the nose, as this is the best place for us to be fully aware of breathing. Attention to the breath as it moves through / at the tip of the nose, like a string between the index fingers and the thumb. We can feel and perceive the string and its movement only at the point of connection of the fingers. Similarly, we perceive internal / nasal breathing movements.

Buddhist authors "Breath after breath" use the analogy of the city gatekeeper: traffic is constantly moving and leaving, but his attention remains alone at the gate. He sees people coming and going, but he doesn't follow anyone. (I think it's as if someone is gently touching a moving belt with their finger: they will feel the movement, but their perception will remain at their fingertips.) Similarly. On our own, we keep our attention at the door of the nose, watching the inhale coming in and the exhale coming out. Naturally, your perception of the tip of your nose and breathing sometimes becomes blurred or distracting, or your attention becomes blurred or dripping. When this happens, just be careful, breathe through your nose, be well aware of the breathing movement at the tip of your nose, and it will refocus your awareness. Feel free to even raise your hand and touch the tip of your nose and make sure your awareness is concentrated there.

Just as our breath becomes pure, so does our consciousness. Sometimes after a period of meditation, we may lose more physical awareness of the tip of the nose and perceive it as a point in front of us, a "point of attention" where the tip of the nose is only the most objective expression.

It is good if we are always aware of the essence and still aware of the movement of the breath there, although its subtle forms may seem more like a train or a flow than the movement of the breath (air), or even a kind of extreme transition of the breath. Because you may know about breathing and not know about the tip of the nose - but you do not know about the tip of the nose and you do not know about breathing - awareness of the tips is the key to effective Anapanasati practice. Also, if we are only aware of breathing, we will only know about physical breathing. But if we are aware of the tip of the nose, we will be aware of the inner breath, more and more subtly, this is the real Breath of Life.

So when you have reached a certain level of breathing meditation, you will find that if you just focus on the tip of your nose, everything else will be in order. Just as closing your eyes eliminates the great activity of brain waves, so focusing on the tip of your nose frees your mind and cuts out random thoughts. At the same time, however, higher possibilities of intuition are included and allow the practitioner to understand deep intuition (vipassana).

Why the tip of the nose?

Language and most languages are unconsciously rooted. That is why we often say things about which we have only excellent knowledge. For example, although very few people believe in (and even few can see) the so-called halo phenomenon - the subtle, colored energy field that surrounds the body - everyone uses an expression. Achievement is related to the aura. When someone is smart, we say he is "bright," and when he is not, we say he is "stupid." When we are cowards, we say they are "yellow". We say that people are "green with jealousy", but jealous people have "blue eyes". If we feel depressed, we say we are "blue," and when we feel very well, we say "pink." When we get angry, we say we "see red." And it is not uncommon to hear about "purple indulgence." All this indicates a subconscious knowledge of the aura. Same with the nose. We talk about people

69

with "nose noses," we call the curious "curious," and we talk about people who are trying to understand something like "looking around." It is said that people with extreme intentions in their work "put their noses in the grinding wheel." All these terms associate the nose with attention and cognition. These statements must be valid because in both Hindu and Buddhist traditions, meditators must pay attention to the tip of the nose. This is obviously of practical importance to provide us with a stable starting point so that our mind does not waver during meditation. But there is much more to this than the faithful meditator will discover. The tip of the nose is the best point for focusing attention and the best for clear perception.

Why that? Because the body is gathered karma. That is, the physical body is an objective manifestation of the karmic forces (energy) created in previous lives - the force that prompted us to incarnate in our bonds. In a sense, the body is a bunch of ignorance, a bunch of nonsense. This is our private network, in which we find ourselves in a helpless trap. By entering this deceptive home during meditation, you run the risk of falling into the subtle energies of karma and becoming more and more connected, even deceived by your wrong paths. Yes, some types of meditation can make us more ignorant and even more enslaved! That is why the Buddha advised Zen as an element of liberation.

There are various energy points and energy sources in the body, which are the vortices of karmic force, the energy mechanisms that support the entire karmic communication system. These centers are powerful accumulators of karmic seeds, and their energy can result in these seeds, leading to more karma. In addition, these centers are home to various "states of consciousness", in fact, nothing but mental hallucinations, poisonous bacteria, and viruses that cause so many samsara diseases. By simply touching these vortices, we will be drawn to them, swaying in their confusion and immersed in their deadly illusion: the dream of death, which we mistakenly call "life."

For this reason, meditation should take place almost outside the body - the tip of the nose is not actually in the body, but where the breath flows (internal release). At least we have to "touch" the body through perception at the tip of the nose because if we focus on a point outside the body, it dissipates our perception and leads to delusions "out of body experience" or simple mental disorientation that ends in deep sleep. When perception is absorbed into the body, Young's principle prevails. When perception is extracted from the body, the principle of yin prevails. But when perception focuses on the tip of the nose during respiratory movements there, both enter a state of perfect equilibrium and at the same time pass in the process of transition from duality to unity.

Thus, the tip of the nose is a gateway to liberated consciousness, as well as a gateway to breathing. After a while, just paying attention to the tip of your nose will turn you into a high consciousness

Thus, the tip of the nose is a gateway to liberated consciousness, as well as a gateway to breathing. After a while, just paying attention to the tip of your nose will turn you into a higher meaning.

When breathing becomes Subtle

The practice of breathing meditation improves breathing and transfers awareness from the outside to the inner breath, from the outer mind to the inner mind, and then to the breath and the meaningless: pure consciousness is the spirit. This process is very similar to the Indian story of a man imprisoned at the top of a tower. To save him, his wife came at night with a scarab, silk thread, cotton rope, rope, and some honey. She tied a string to one of the beetle's hind legs, dropped a drop of honey on its horn, and then placed it on the wall of the tower directly in the window where her husband was waiting. Desiring honey, the dung beetle crawled forward, always moving forward until it reached the window, and the prisoner, who removed the rope, held the beetle. Then the wife tied the string to the silk thread, and the husband drew it up. Finally, she tied the rope to the end of the string, and he pulled it up, fastened it, and then climbed out freely. In this parable, everything goes from subtle to coarse, but in Anapanasati breathing goes from coarse to subtle - and free.

Although breathing becomes clearer, it is good when you observe it (perhaps it is more accurate to say that your perception becomes pure, although breathing becomes lighter in nature) You still do not need to do it consciously, because your own attention will improve it. Attention is key.

When breathing is "lost"

When you "lose" the consciousness of breathing because it becomes too thin, you can do one of two things: 1) Take one or more deep breaths through your nose (close your mouth) to restore consciousness. about breathing, and then continue to watch him as usual. 2) Be aware of the tip of your nose (touch it if necessary), and just watch what is happening there - or not - what is happening. Usually, in just a few seconds, this will allow you to feel the subtle movement of breathing again, but otherwise, you can just sit and be aware of the tip of your nose - seemingly no breath. Over time, you will experience the perception of fine breathing, and you will be able to continue to observe it as usual. This is because the very tip of the nose is an ideal sensor for delicate breathing movements.

When nothing seems to be happening, don't force anything. Just keep your consciousness on the tip of your nose: watch, look, Over time, very subtle breathing will be noticed there. No need to force, just watch.

# Chapter 7: Guided Meditation To Boost Positivity

It is important to get rid of any unnecessary attachments.

Unimportant attachments are things you no longer need.

These things will make you feel miserable and prevent you from achieving your goals of living a happy life. This is a key factor in your future success. To achieve that position, it is important to let go of all things that could bring you down. It is important to remember that anyone can be anything.

There are people in our lives who will always try to bring us down. These people fear your success in life.

They will do everything they can to bring you down, regardless of how positive you try to be. You need to get moving and rid yourself of them like the plague. You must choose to live, and not just live.

You must refuse to accept any and all limitations that may be holding you back.

This being said, I wish you to use this affirmation daily. You will see the benefits of practice and it will become a habit when you train.

You are enough as you are. It is important to let go of the demon idea that you can compare yourself with others. To be specific and stay focused, you need to have success standards. Once you have established these standards, you can set your goals and objectives. Your vision should be related to your life's mission. These are the foundations of your success.

You can judge yourself according to the rules and regulations that you have created in your success criteria. You are enough just the way that you were born. There is no part of yourself that isn't there. Never compare yourself to others.

Affirmation can help you realize your worthiness. In a matter of minutes, you can control your body image. It will also help you achieve some personal goals, such as a healthy body.

Your purpose must be fulfilled. Your existence should be known by the world, and you should be prepared to demonstrate your accomplishments. Positive actions that will lead to success are key to showing the world your accomplishments. People who are trendsetting are often our trend-setters.

Because they have done something good or bad, they are a popular trend. They are then well-known all over the globe. You must remember to be positive in order to receive this motivational affirmation.

It is important to set the standard for what you can offer and be an inspiration for others. You must sweep until the president stops his journey to congratulate anyone who has been assigned to you. To be happy and successful, you must strive to achieve your highest potential. This affirmation reminds us that no one can stop you from achieving or fulfilling your purpose in our lives. This thought will help you get to where you want to go. Focus on what you want to achieve and don't let anyone stop you.

It is important to be results-oriented. You must keep your eyes on the prize in every aspect of your life. You should always be focused on your results. This is how you can maximize your productivity.

You must create space for success in order to achieve this. Your life will be more successful. Avoid making excuses for failure that could damage your reputation and lower your success rate. These phrases will bring you joy every day. There is no need to make excuses for not being able to accomplish something. You can be yourself and continue to work until you achieve your goals. This is how your mind will settle and give you peace of mind. You will be able to live a stress-free life. This will show in your body image.

You have the power to make your happiness a reality. Happiness is a quality of life that can inspire positive emotions and feelings.

It's like a gear that is geared toward your successful life. It is important to stay positive. To do this, you need to take charge of your happiness. Being responsible is a virtue. It will help you be brave enough to take on any situation.

Your joy is the key to your success. No one should interfere with it. Be happy and responsible for your happiness.

No one should make you mad. Angriness can only cause you to feel emotional emotions that will ultimately affect your life and your body image. This should have convinced you to accept this affirmation. Use it to open your mornings and make a habit of it throughout your day.

You can achieve weight loss success by focusing on areas that provide you with clear visions of affirmations. Beliefs are powerful phrases that can bring about positivity and are not to be confused with affirmations. These affirmations will help you stay focused, positive, and relaxed. There are many affirmations to choose from. Pick the ones that you are comfortable with and get into a routine to make them permanent. You will notice a significant drop in your weight.

The album also encourages you to be positive about yourself. It is a world of motivation. This is why motivational affirmations can help you achieve your ultimate goal and bring more happiness and relaxation to your life. These phrases are explained in detail in this episode. I hope that you prefer a beautiful body full of happiness and pleasure. You can live a happy life because you've followed the principles and implemented them fully.

You must live a happy, healthy life. A vital life is one that inspires happiness and encourages you to live positively and happily. These actions result in inner peace and blessings. You must practice affirmative self-control in order to achieve all of these. You will be able to control everything around you.

This album contains many aspects of life you should be following no matter what. This will allow you to be clear and direct about your life, and prevent obesity from becoming a problem. I am glad you found this episode about hypnosis for weight loss important. This area will explain how important these exercises are, particularly in your personal life. This album provides the right guidelines you should follow. Meditation can be used to lose weight, particularly if you follow hypnosis exercises. Grab this album now and get started as soon as you can.

Meditation for Weight Loss serves as a guideline to help you reduce your weight. It is your responsibility to read it carefully and follow every step. It is important to know how you can set smart goals that are easily achievable. This will ensure that you have a happy and fulfilled life. This is why it's important to take care of this album and make every episode count towards your weight loss goals.

I believe this album has been a blessing to you. Please, check out the following sites. Do not hesitate to mention its significance or importance to readers looking for easy ways to lose weight.

When it comes to our patterns of thought, symbolism is a big topic. When you are hungry, you might think "I'm starving," or "I'm sick," but these are powerful statements that come to mind because of how our brains work. To better understand things, we connect thoughts. As a way of figuring things out, we also make absolute statements. It's possible to fail in a diet once and then think "I can't make this." Our brains create these assumptions because it's how we come up with solutions.

This is why we need to change our thinking and instead wire our brains to think positively. Use the "I can," I will," and "I will" statements to create affirmations. You can use "I" in all affirmations you make, as this is about increasing your positivity, creativity, and not for someone else.

Once you have used the "I" phrases, you can then make a definite statement. You should never describe what you don't have. Also, you should avoid pointing out flaws even if you are positive. Use strong absolutes. The area where you have the most difficulty is the one that you should add the most affirmations to.

# Chapter 8: Mantra Meditation

We will start with the definition. The mantra could be a Sanskrit term, which may derive from two roots: man (meaning mind or think) and safe (or to try with means/equipment). Mantras can be described as tools for the mind, or tools to liberate your mind.

Mantras can be translated into some literal meanings. Most mantras remain true to tradition, with their value derived mainly from their sound quality. Some words are very short and only one-syllable. Some are longer and contain many words.

What is Mantra Meditation Mantra meditation?

Sometimes, the mantra can be recited. Sometimes it is recited. It is sometimes repeated quickly, but it can also be repeated slowly at other times. It is sometimes repeated by oneself.

What's the purpose of the mantra in meditation?

The mantra acts as a focus. It acts as a distraction to the monkey-mind and helps it become more calm and focused. It functions in a similar way to your breathing or another meditation object during this sense.

A mantra can also be used to transform your consciousness. This aspect of mantra meditation is more complex than others, so it might not be for everyone. It teaches that each sound and vibration is only one quality. It can provide the different states of mind, consciousness, and energy when it is needed again.

MANTRAS REQUIRE ATTENTION

SOUND TRANSFORMATIVE MPOWER

You might ask, "What is so special about repeating one word?" It is a powerful tool for meditation.

Sound is a mixture. Every cell of your body vibrates. Every cell in the universe vibrates to its own rhythm. Your thoughts and emotions are vibrations within your body and consciousness.

Sound patterns can also impact your body's hydration, hormone secretion and cognition.

It is possible to see your mind, or psyche, as a collection of patterns that vibrate at a different frequency, speed, volume, and frequency. Yoga and mystics have found that if you keep a certain sound vibration at a given time, your mind and body can often be transformed.

It can be used for emotional changes, such as anxiety, pain relief, mood enhancement, and mood improvement. It can be used to control your mind and reach deeper levels of consciousness.

Every musician and filmmaker will tell you how sound can evoke emotions, thoughts, or moods. Imagine meditating on a song that can change your perspective or help you heal. With care and attention, imagine this programming feature in your brain.

Your body, thoughts and emotions are affected by sound, rhythm and speech. Mantra meditation employs the three elements that purify and soothe your mind and heart.

Mantra, an instrument of the mind can be used to bring about profound changes in your body and psyche, and alter your consciousness. Mantra meditation is a method of moving your consciousness around a sound and amplifying it to achieve maximum effect. Mantra meditation is a popular method of yoga contemplation. It is considered the easiest and most secure.

Mantra Thoughts Often, we are focused on one thing at a time. Multitasking is a quick way to change the focus of our attention. Multitasking can be taxing and ineffective.

The implication of this is simple for meditation: When you pay attention solely to the mantra, other thoughts, memories or sensations are not interfering with your focus. Imagine that you can string two mantras together and then, at the end, you switch to the next one. This will allow you to meditate in a peaceful and beautiful place for the entire duration.

One mantra can replace 10,000 ideas from one thought. It is the concept that brings peace and awareness. This will allow you to unify your scattered attention and make it more powerful.

Meditation is the same process as meditation with other objects of concentration like breathing or visual events. A mantra has the advantage of easily overriding mental speech which is for many the dominant form of conscious thought.

The mantra's rhythmic nature also helps to overcome the annoying songs that pop up during meditation. These are some of those things that do not happen as quickly in other forms of meditation.

This lesson outlines some studies that show how chanting mantras can increase concentration, well-being and resistance to negative inputs.

Meditation Mantra Meditation Necessary to Mantra (How To Choose) Your attitude towards meditation, whether spiritual or secular, will determine which mantra you choose. You can also influence the results of your practice.

However, some mantras can be used in both directions and are universal. The Sanskrit mantra Om followed by Ham is one example.

You can use your native language to create a mantra. This is often a sentence or a word that conveys a message to your subconscious.

These are my suggestions for choosing a word.

The most important thing is meaning. You should choose a word or sentence that represents something you are looking to improve, feel better, or connect with. You can choose love, peace and freedom, awareness, light and courage, or any combination thereof.

Continue reading. The sound of the word must be spoken. This is the only way to feel this. Repeat it for a few times and notice how you feel afterwards.

Avoid words with ambiguous meanings and potentially negative connotations.

There are many mantras you can choose from before you decide on the one that resonates with your most. Let's say you need a mantra to calm your anxiety. Om has a calming effect and you will probably enjoy using it.

It is better to choose a similar mantra once you have selected it. This will help create its effect.

A mantra can be used to thank someone for helping you achieve a spiritual goal. Every word has its "energy," which is consumed by the way it's repeated. It is wise to choose a standard mantra, a word or sound that spiritual seekers have used for hundreds of years with an indifferent attitude.

It is possible to be more happy using the first word in the language it was discovered (usually Sanskrit or Pali, Hebrew, Aramaic or Tibetan). It is important to correctly pronounce and pronounce the mantra, since we want to repeat the specific sound vibration.

First, decide what spiritual tradition or lineage speaks to your heart. Once you have identified what your echo is best, you can move on to the next step.

Talk to someone who is a teacher in that tradition and ask for a mantra. Ask for ideas. Ask for suggestions.

You can research the mantras that are used on that particular path and then try them all for a few days to determine which one is most helpful in your quest.

As a spiritual practice, you should try to think about the meaning and situation of a mantra. This is why mantra meditation can be a powerful practice for affirming your glory.

A mantra can be described as a password, key, a specific state of consciousness or universal principle that you wish to experience.

This approach requires you to keep your mantra secret. This mantra is available online and is used by thousands of people. It is the sacred secret. If you keep your mantra secret, it will have a deeper effect on your consciousness.

Level and progress

Repeating a mantra repeatedly will increase its "activation" or "magnetization. For one-word mantras, it is believed that after 125,000 repetitions, it "gets its own lifetime." It charges itself with a repeated meditation mantra. When the mantra is the most powerful thought in the mind, you can then consider it to bring about peace.

When your mantra gains momentum, repetition becomes easier. It's almost like we just "start" or log in to the mantra and it continues on its own, leading to internal silence.

This is a common progression in practice.

Oral recitation: You say it aloud. You can engage more of your senses and stay focused.

Whispering – Lips and tongue move but there isn't much sound. This is subtler than oral recitation and makes a more powerful sound.

Mental recitation: You only need to repeat the mantra in your head. There is some movement in the throat and tongue at the beginning. These movements fade over time and the practice becomes purely mental. This is the normal phase of mantra cultivation.

Spontaneous Listening - While you may not be repeating the mantra right now, the mantra is moving in your head, automatically, all the time. It doesn't matter how loud or fast it is. It is natural to want to be repeated, so it doesn't matter if it is heard repeatedly. This level is known as Jaap Japan, and it is silent mantra meditation.

As you can see there has been progress from the unpolished to the subtle, evolution to effortlessness. One mistake people make is to try to lower levels and start with a mental recurrence, or a spontaneous repetition. In a way, it is more difficult than making step-by-step steps.

Even if oral recitation is not your thing and you need to travel on an emotional level, I recommend that you start with just a few rounds of whispering in the beginning. This will help you focus more on the mantra.

No matter where you are on the scale, if your mind becomes distracted by the mantra, in thinking, or sleeping, you can take it down one notch. You can make a conscious effort to keep it going until you are able to carry it one more time.

A mantra can be combined with other practices such as visualization or devotion that specialize in a particular cycle, devotion, or other areas. These primary techniques are often practiced with a secular/agnostic outlook. However, some of them have metaphysics.

The guidelines below outline the basic principles of meditation with the Dhyana mantra. They also apply to all other practices.

Asana mudra is a method of meditation for ceremonial mantras.

You can practice the mantra with informal practice by repeating it in your head, while you do other things. This is a great way to say thank you for focusing on your life.

You can vary the speed at which you recite the mantra, depending on how long it is. The shorter episodes (1-3 syllables) are more common than the longer phrases.

It is important to remember that mantras and techniques are often very specific. If you don't have one, try different repetition speeds to find what works best for you.

I found that both fast and slow repetitions of the mantra led to silence. The "taste" of silence can be different for each person. When you repeat it slowly, it feels like you are in a deep, zooming-in, and theta waves feel like silence. It is intense and "in flux" when recited quickly. Gamma-waves are silent when recited slowly.

It is better to keep the pace steady and not change it multiple times throughout the session.

Loudness and force

If you are a boisterous thinker, it is a good idea to increase the volume of the mantra's repetition. This can make it more loud and thicker. Your attention may drift off to a tangent without thinking.

When your mind is calmer, the mantra can often become "thinner" and "lower," similar to a high-frequency sound you barely hear. The mantra is more like a sound vibration than the word itself, as it almost loses its meaning.

Let it happen if this is something that comes naturally to you. If you forget the mantra, it is best to get it back up to a point where you are able to stick to it.

You have a few options, regardless of whether or not you are able to coordinate your mantra with your breathing.

Both exhalation and inhalation. You can repeat your mantra once while you breathe in and then again when you exhale. You can also increase your speed and repeat the mantra 3 times while you breathe in and 3 times when you exhale. Or, you can do it repeatedly if it suits your breathing rate and length. You can also say half of your mantra when you inhale, then the other half when you exhale.

Only exhale. Repeat the mantra, exhaling with no voice.

You don't have to pay attention to your breath if you are required to breathe. Living naturally with the mantra will eventually become a rhythm.

The mind's function, whether you are reciting it or just meditating on the mantra, is to focus on each repetition. Every replay should be fresh, new, and full of life and awareness.

The mantra will unite your thoughts. It is your mantra. Give it every ounce of attention. This can be made easier by using some mantras such as care, curiosity reverence gratitude or any other appropriate exercises.

Your mind is the antenna and the mantra is a station. The problem with this antenna is the fact that it switches frequencies automatically. We want to keep the antenna in sync and consistent with the mantra.

After some time, you will see that there is more to your mind than just one layer of thinking. Move your awareness to a deeper level.

Do not force your thoughts. Tension can lead to tension which can be detrimental to meditation. It is important to keep the awareness of the mantra in your mind, and not become overwhelmed moment by moment. It is a constant, relaxed awareness.

Many passages in yoga contemplation tradition include mantra meditation. These practices often include mantra repetition, breathing, specific visualization, contemplation and chakras.

The practice of reciting mantras, called Chakras, in certain lineages (Kundalini Yoga and Rhythm Yoga, Tantra Yoga), focusing on particular chakras (centers) within the body, is known as Chakra Yoga. This can be done by repeatedly repeating the sound of each chakra's seed. These are the majority of the chakra mantras. The pronunciation guide is in parentheses.

Tantra, yoga, and other schools of yoga have synchronizing mantras that are accompanied by specific breathing patterns. Here are some examples of yoga mantras.

A-HAM mantra ("I am"). Repetition "A" after exhalation, and "HAM" after exhalation.

SO-HAM Mantra Repeat the "SO" and "HAM" mantras on exhalation. This will bring your attention up and down your spine.

Soham - Hama. You can inhale through the left nostril and repeat "such", then exhale through the right nostril, repeating "ham".

Now, exhale through your left nostril while inhaling "ham" through the right nostril. Next, repeat the process by inhaling "ham" through the right nostril. This is a continuous cycle. You should take at least ten courses.

You can do many other complicated exercises but they will not be as useful if you prefer simplicity.

Rituals and Visualization

Mantras Yoga school makes extensive use of mantras, visualizations and rituals. This topic is beyond the scope this lesson.

Contribution

Vedanta (Jnana Yoga), mantras that are used to grasp spiritual truth, is used. These mantras are known as "Mahasaya", or great. These are the highest:

Ahom Brahmasmi ("I am Brahma")

Tatami Asi ("You're art")

SIRVA Kalevala Brahma (All is Brahmi): In this practice, meditation is about contemplating the meaning of the mantra rather than reciting words or sounds. It is a way to increase knowledge and understanding.

Writes mantras (chanting of Lakshita).

You can use this practice to increase your senses by writing mantras and watching mantras. These are the basics:

For the practice of truthfulness, separate a notebook and pencil/pen.

Write the mantra down on paper and repeat it throughout the session.

Try to be as concise and neat as possible in order to speed up the process. This might require greater concentration.

Keep your eyes fixed on the notebook. Until you are done with the session, do not move them.

Deity Meditation – Tantra and Bhakti Marg Pasages

Both these meditations are done with open eyes. 108 beads of beads, also known as garlands, are used to increase repetition.

The actual Tantra was developed in India and Lamaism. It is very different from the Tantra that is popularized in the West. This Tantra aims to enhance sexual function.

Yoga is the main cultivation deity in the tradition of tantra. The practice seeks to attain a state that allows one to feel a sense of unity with the universal forces of nature. This can be used to awaken spiritual insight and other qualities. Jungian psychologists refer to these deities in this way: they are fanatics of collective unconscious.

The mantra is the vehicle for this purpose. The mantra in Tantra is not prayer. It is not the name of the deity but the sound-form. When we can relate to the mantra's convenience the vibration of our mind becomes connected to the larger sense. This is itself a characteristic a vibratory nature.

Tantra (Hindu, Buddhist) is a practice that allows the practitioner to use one or more exercises in addition to repeating the mantra.

a-Imagine the form of the chosen deity.

b-Include the attributes of that deity (power, beauty, knowledge, etc. .

c-Even when you gaze upon the symbol or image (yantras) of the deity.

d-Feelings that are filled with reverence, wonder, devotion, or devotion towards the deity.

e-Develop a mindset of identification with the deity through the mantra.

The famous shakti seeds are examples of tantric mantras: aim, haim and scrim; haleem.

Bhakti Yoga's mantra is repeated repeatedly by the practitioner with feelings of devotion as a prayer.

These are examples of Hindu mantras that are popular for Hindu deities in the Hindu pantheon.

Om Namath Shivaya -> Shiva

Vishnu -> Om Namo Bhagavata Vasudevaya

Ganesh -> Om Gam Ganapataye Namaha

Saraswati -> Maa Saraswati Namah In

The mantra is used more in Buddhism to focus the mind.

Some mantras in Theravada are used to aid concentration, particularly by people. The venerable Azan Smedho suggests the mantra Budo. This is the "Bud", which we recommend that you inhale and then exhale, for the complete cycle of the mental cycle.

Mahayana has many mantras that are associated with different types of Buddha. This mantra can be used to meditate, but chanting can also be found in many Buddhist traditions, such as Zen.

Reciting Nam Myoho Renge Kyo, Nikiren Buddhists' most important practice, is their main focus.

Here's a list with Buddhist mantras that can be used for meditation.

Pali Mantra

Sabby Satta Sukhi Hotu

Om Shanti

Buddha Gadhafi

Charanam. Dammam Sarana Panchami. Sangha Sarana Panchami.

Sanskrit Mantra

Gate Paragate Parasamgate Body Sova

Om Mani Padme Hum

Om Tare Tuttare Sourav

Chinese

Namo Amitofo

Christian Mantra Meditation

Prayer, also known as Christian meditation or Christian prayer, is equivalent to mantra meditation. The Christian tradition will choose a holy word and it is then repeated with feelings devotion.

Here are some examples Christian mantras: God Father, Jesus, Mary Abba Mercy, Love or Maranatha (Aramaic meaning "Come Lord!" "

It is important to note that this form of Christian meditation was developed by John Main, an Irish Benedictine monk who studied mantra meditation from a Hindu master during his time in Malaysia.

Transcendental meditation

TM is perhaps the most popular type of mantra meditation in India. Despite all the marketing efforts to separate them, the TM method is essentially a type of mantra meditation.

You can find the official story on their website. I can however, turn your attention away from it. This is not a summary of facts.

Their technique is mantra meditation. This can be done without having to spend a lot of money.

They do not teach the same mantras to every student, but they are supported by their gender or age. Here's a list of TM mantras.

Although the TM organization is secular, they have deep spiritual roots. This is why the Gurus are able to descend through the initiation ceremony.

They often teach that the TM technique doesn't require effort. As we have discussed, giving up all action and just focusing on the mantra are two of the things that can be done effectively after a long period of coaching.

With awareness and focus, we have achieved the same objective. You can quickly reach a plateau if you just forget about it and continue to practice. Although it can lead to a pleasant state of relaxation and rest, this is not likely to result in deep concentration or samadhi.

Positively, many people can start a meditation practice and market it to others through the TM organization. If you are a TM practitioner and find it acceptable, don't be discouraged by my writing. You can continue the process.

You can change your method if you don't have too many problems.

Chapter 10: Navigating Chakra Yoga

The first step in chakra yoga is to identify your blockages and then learn which sequences and poses balance them. This will inform your practice, and help you to create a structured and guided approach that is more effective at healing you. Once you've decided on what you want to concentrate on, you can put together a plan that will guide you in achieving your goals.

You may also notice imbalances in several chakras as you get more in touch with yourself. It is tempting to try everything at once, but it is best to be careful. It is better to concentrate on one thing at the time, as with all things. While you may be able to move through yoga sequences that address different chakras, it is best to focus on one thing at a time. For example, if your goal is to unlock your root chakra, you can start by focusing your energy there.

There are seven major chakras. Because it lies at the base of the spine, the root chakra is the most important. It acts as the foundation for all the other chakras. It is best to balance multiple chakras at once. This will cause a ripple effect, as healing moves up the spine, creating a solid foundation that allows all chakras to heal.

You should practice at least once per week. You can practice every day if you are able. You can start with just one session, and then add more sessions as you progress. Because of the feeling you get afterward, you will want to increase your sessions.

Create Your Own Practice

You are likely looking for a way to create a yoga routine and practice at home. It is possible to create a yoga area in your home that encourages regular practice. It should be visually appealing and calm for you. This space should encourage creativity and help you to be more creative. You don't need a place to store your yoga props in your home. Instead, keep them in a safe place. This will help you feel more comfortable when you use them.

I'll be covering the essential yoga props in more detail later. But first, I want to mention how it is great to have your own yoga mat. Your yoga mat is your sacred space, where you can heal your body, mind, and spirit. It must be cleaned and maintained in a safe manner. People often use public mats in their gym or studio where they take classes. This is an excellent option for those who are limited on space, but it is not the best choice if your goal is to create a personal chakra practice and heal yourself. I strongly encourage you to purchase and care for your yoga mat.

You will discover that your yoga mat is the center of your practice as you develop it. It has been my yoga mat for five years and is still going strong. Its dusty pink color makes me smile every time I see it. The material also feels great on my skin. My mat is a friend and a close companion. It strengthens the special relationship you have with yoga and your mat.

You can bond with your practice by setting up a yoga space. But it is also important to create a routine. You can use this as motivation to continue your practice. Setting goals is essential in every aspect of your life. Setting goals will allow you to establish your practice and keep you motivated to return to your mat.

LISTEN TO YOUR BODY

This book will take you step by step through the various yoga sequences and poses to help you make the right choices when performing the asanas. While this book will help you with your practice, it cannot replace a personal yoga teacher or your knowledge about your body. You can always move out of a pose if you are having trouble or feeling uneasy. Modifications and yoga props can be used to make the pose more comfortable for you. Use your body as a guide, and listen to it. It is good to push yourself to learn and improve. However, forcing yourself into yoga poses you aren't ready for is not the best way to go. You can work your way up to the full expression of the poses. Be patient with yourself.

It is important that you recognize the difference between good and bad pain. This is because it helps you to get stronger. Sharp pain is experienced in the joints (where two bones are joined). You should immediately get out of that pose. As your muscles relax and become more flexible, dull pain in the middle is normal. You can trust your body's signals. It is up to you to understand the messages.

Poses to Hold

While I will give a time limit for each pose in a sequence in this book, it is important to listen and decide for yourself. You will develop an intuition about the length of each pose as you practice yoga more regularly and deepen your practice.

You should hold the poses for at least three to five deep, full breaths. You will need to hold the poses longer for a yin (or restorative) practice. This means that you should hold them for three to five minutes. These aren't hard-and-fast rules. Sometimes, your teacher, or the yoga instructor you're following, may suggest that you hold a particular pose for a longer time to emphasize a movement or to move through a pose faster. It all depends on the style of the class, the theme or purpose of the sequence and the teacher.

Your body can also send signals to your brain to tell you when it's time to get out of a pose. You will need to pay attention to your body to understand what types of pain you are experiencing. Understanding that not all pain is bad is essential to your growth. Your body will always choose the path of least resistance. If you are unsure, don't feel the pain. You can always get out of it if you need to until you have a better understanding of what you should be feeling. You will eventually gain wisdom, so be patient and practice consistently and regularly.

LEAVE YOUR COMFORT ZONE

Yoga practitioners often talk about finding your "edge" and putting your body in that pose before you get out. As you practice yoga, you will discover more about your own personal edge. Understanding when your body's survival mode kicks in is a good way to determine where that edge is. This is when your body gets tired and chooses the path of least resistance. When you recognize that the discomfort or pain you feel isn't the worst kind of pain, and are able stay in the pose without causing any harm to your body and mind, you can then acknowledge your edge and move on.

Your body will improve, become stronger, and have more flexibility when you move beyond your edge. You also notice a change in the energy flow to your chakras. You must make changes to restore balance to your chakras, particularly if there is a blockage. This will be something you learn over the course of your own personal journey. Be patient and trust yourself.

Harnessing Your Breath

Your breath is an important aspect of yoga. It can be used to move through the poses and also as a support tool. You can use specific breathing exercises and techniques to relax, increase energy, feel grounded and gain energy. You can also incorporate breathing into your asana practice to improve your postures and your overall health.

Your breath is the life force of your body. Therefore, "prana," or "breath," can all be interchangeably used. Although there is some difference between energy (or breath) in terms of location and physicality, it is the same thing. Breath is the intake or release of energy. Inhaling brings energy and power into the body, which continues to flow through the chakras and throughout the body. Inhaling allows you to exhale and continues the flow of energy.

If you are anxious, breathing can help you relax and slow down your heartbeat. You can also use it to stretch deeper. You can exhale to gently ease your body into the stretch. During meditation, you can use your breath to communicate with your subconscious. Focusing on your breath can help you pay attention to your body's movements and allow you to feel inside. You will develop a deeper connection with your breath and learn more about your body.

GRANTHIS (KNOTS)

Granthi, which means "knot", refers to the idea that blocked energy can be restrictive and hard to untie. Granthis are the most common cause of blocked chakras. They can block prana's flow throughout the body. These can cause you to become stuck in your own ways and prevent you from being open to new possibilities. These may be more general or more specific depending on where the granthi is located and the cause. These are some of the ways you can release your granthis. You can also incorporate them into your chakra practice.

BANDHAS (LOCKS).

The bandhas (or locks) can be used to help you release your granthis and unblock your chakras. Bandhas can help you move prana from areas where it is blocked by chakra blocks or granthis to other parts of your body. You can incorporate four bandhas into your chakra yoga practice.

1. Mula Bandha. This is the root lock. To activate it, squeeze in the muscles at Muladhara's first chakra. This is also known as a Kegel and is used to strengthen the vaginal muscles prior and after childbirth.

2. Uddiyana Bandha. This lock is located in your abdominal region. It involves the act of drawing your organs upward as you bend forward. As you bring those organs and muscles up, your hands can rest on your legs.

3. Jalandhara Bandha. This lock is located in the neck area. You can achieve this by sitting tall with your legs crossed and your hands on your legs. Your sternum and chin should meet at the halfway point.

These bandhas can be practiced and held for as long time as you're able. This will help you to become stronger and increase the flow of energy throughout your body.

RELEASE YOUR PAST

Sometimes past traumas and tensions may be brought to the surface when we open our chakras and balance them. To avoid experiencing pain, many of us suppress painful and traumatic experiences from our past. As I said, our bodies and minds tend to choose the path of least resistance. Sometimes, avoiding emotional pain can be a part of that path.

It may be easier to avoid pain than to feel it, but it is important that we accept it and persevere so we can move on. Take the time to observe any feelings that arise during chakra yoga. It is okay to cry. Don't be afraid to express your emotions and let them out. Journaling can be used to help you get rid of your thoughts and feelings.

After you have observed your thoughts and emotions, you can recognize that what you are seeing is not real. It is merely a memory. Recognize that thoughts and feelings are not yours. They don't define you. You can observe them without judgement before they fade away. Although it may take some time before you feel better, you should not allow those feelings to return. Before you move on, make sure to properly release them and

use observation, journaling and emotional
release to do so.

# Chapter 9: Retreats And Community

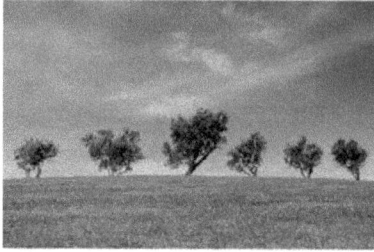

You've presently taken in a portion of the rudiments of reflection. You can keep on rehearsing these strategies at home. Day by day contemplation is useful for the body and cerebrum and can be accomplished by anybody.

If you feel prepared to make the following stride, at that point joining a network reflection gathering or in any event, heading off to a retreat could be a phenomenal decision.

Network contemplations focuses are regularly extremely steady and empowering of the thoughtful excursion. It's an occasion to meet like-minded individuals, get tips, and address individuals who are further along on their excursion or even assist pristine apprentices to locate the

correct posture or reflection style. The middle may offer guided reflections, where one individual leads a gathering. This isn't something that can be accomplished at home when it's only you all alone. Sound contemplations, for example, gong treatment is likewise something that requires a subsequent individual. Is likewise the ideal spot to learn further developed techniques, for example, strolling contemplations or reflective yoga.

If there is nothing similar to this close by, a smart thought could be to shape a little reflection hover yourself with various companions, neighbors, and local people. To do this, organize a huge space inside your home, cleaning up encompassing regions and covering nosy pictures or articles. Pads should dissipate over the floor, ideally, there should be an assortment of shadings. Recollect what we found out about shading impacts in the past sections? A few participants may wish to sit on a particular shaded pad to improve their experience. Choose among yourselves on the off chance that you'd incline toward guided or individual quiet reflection. Whenever guided contemplation is best, one individual can lead, or a care disc can be played.

If you work extended periods of time in an office, why not set up a little room far removed for you and your partners to have short contemplation meetings at lunch? Your supervisor might be agreeably shocked at the amount more gainful the evenings become.

A retreat is typically a more expanded and focussed method of encountering the power of meditation. It tends to be host to numerous individuals for anyplace between a day and a while. Contemplations will be organized for the duration of the day, from promptly toward the beginning of the day to nightfall, with no strain to focus on a base number of sittings. Each retreat has a bunch of rules which should be perused before making a booking. Some may offer end of the week bundles or serious-entire days. On the off chance that you don't have any

duties at home, you may even want to participate in half a month to progress colossally, both profoundly and actually.

A retreat is frequently quiet or calm, and could likewise offer workshops and occasions to go to meetings with prepared experts and priests. The quietness of the room is supporting and healthy, quite a welcome help from a world loaded with TVs and cell phones. Indeed, even the dinners are ordinarily knowledgeable about an absolutely careful way, with complete consideration applied to the way toward tasting and gulping, flavors, and tones.

If you need to start stirring up your contemplation experience, why not take a cover and pad to an extensive outside territory, away from groups, and endeavor an open-air meeting? This will contrast significantly to your home setting, with new and irregular sounds, scents, and sensations. Practice care to inundate yourself in the manner the breeze feels on your cheeks, how the feathered creatures sing to each other, how the blossoms smell, what the grass feels like underneath your legs. Does the air feel distinctive when you inhale it in? Is it colder? Fresher?

In conclusion, start to develop the expertise of contemplating anyplace. Start little, for example, a recreation center seat in a canine strolling region, so passers-by are available yet not really problematic. The seashore makes for a magnificent tactile encounter and tests the constraints of fixation. Recall that thinking isn't tied in with purchasing devices and instruments or requiring 'things', it is something that you heft around within you – a capacity – that can be utilized and delighted in whenever, anyplace.

# Chapter 10: Desire - Food - Sex

All ordinary vital movements are not related to our true being and come from outside; they do not belong to the soul and do not arise in it, but are waves of the common Nature, Prakriti.

Desires come from outside, enter the subconscious vital and rise to the surface of consciousness. We are aware of them only when they reach the surface and the mind becomes aware of them. Desires seem to us to be ours because we feel them ascending from the vital into the mind and do not know that they have come from outside.

It is not the desire itself that belongs to our vital being, as well as makes it react, not the desire itself, but the habit of responding to the waves or currents of suggestion coming from universal Prakriti.

In essence, to reject desire means to reject the element of craving, to put it outside the brackets of consciousness as an alien element, not belonging to your true self and inner nature. But the refusal to indulge in suggestions of desire is also part of the rejection; abstinence from the suggested action, if this action is wrong, should be part of yogic practice.

It can be called suppression only when the refusal is carried out incorrectly, through some mental ascetic principle or strict moral norm. The difference between suppression and essential inner rejection is the difference between mental or moral control and spiritual cleansing.

When you live in true consciousness, you feel the desires outside yourself, you feel how they enter the mind and vital parts from the outside, from the universal lower Prakriti. Under normal conditions, a person does not feel this; people begin to be conscious of desire only when it is already there, when it has penetrated inside and found shelter or habitual refuge, and therefore they think that this desire is their own, that it is a part of themselves.

Therefore, the first condition for getting rid of desire is to become conscious with true consciousness; for it becomes much easier to reject desire in this case than when you have to fight with it as a part of yourself that must be expelled from your being. It is easier to throw off a growth than to cut off what we feel as part of our flesh.

It is easier to get rid of desire also when the soul being comes to the fore; for in the psychic being as such there are no desires, in it there are only aspirations, as well as the search for the Divine and love for him, as well as for everything connected with him. The constantly felt presence of a soul being itself causes the emergence of true consciousness and almost involuntarily corrects the movements of your nature.

DEMAND AND DESIRE

Demand and desire are just two sides of the same thing, and in the case of desire, the feeling does not necessarily have to be agitated or disturbed; on the contrary, desire can be quietly rooted and constant, or it can quietly return again and again.

The demand or desire comes from the mind or vital, and the soul or spiritual need is something else entirely. The soul does not demand and does not want, it strives; it entrusts itself without putting forward any conditions, and does not turn away when its striving does not find a response immediately, for the soulful completely trusts the Divine or the Guru, and can wait for the due hour or the descent of Divine Grace.

Perseverance is characteristic of the soul, but it exerts its pressure not on the Divine, but on nature, highlighting with its light all the shortcomings that block the path to comprehension, filtering out everything mixed, ignorant or imperfect in the experience or movements of Yoga and never satisfied with itself or existing nature, while will not make her completely open to the Divine, free from all forms of ego, self-denying, simple and true in her position and all her movements.

This is what must be firmly established in the mind, vital and physical consciousness before the supramentalisation of the whole nature is possible. Otherwise, what you gain turns out to be more or less brilliant insights and experiences on the mental, vital and physical plane, which are half shedding light and half confusing, being inspired by some larger mind or vital, or at best, from the mental spheres that lie above the person, mediating between the intellect and the Over-mind.

Up to a certain point, all this can be very stimulating and satisfying a person, and it is good for those who wish to receive some kind of spiritual attainment on these planes; but the supramental comprehension is something much more difficult and exacting in terms of the conditions of realization, and the most difficult of all is to ensure its descent to the physical level.

It takes a long time to get rid of desire completely. But if you can immediately separate it from your nature and become aware of it as a force that comes from outside and throws claws into the vital and physical, it will be easier to get rid of this occupier. You're too used to feeling him as part of yourself or as something grafted on you, which makes it harder for you to deal with his movements and end his old control over you.

You should rely mainly, first and foremost, on the Power of the Mother and on nothing else, no matter how useful it may seem. The Sun and Light can and will help if it is the true Light and the true Sun, but they are not able to take the place of the Mother's Force.

The sadhak should have as few basic necessities as possible; for there is only very little that you really cannot do without in life. Everything else either makes life easier, or decorates it, or serves as a luxury item. The yogi has the right to possess or enjoy such things only in two cases:

(i) If he uses them in the SADHANA solely for the exercise of possession without attachment or desire and learns to apply them correctly - in accordance with Divine Will, treating them appropriately, with proper organization, care and application, or

(ii) if he has already achieved true freedom from desire and attachment, so that the loss, deprivation or absence of such things does not touch him in the least and does not affect him in the least. If some thirst, desire, demand or claim to possess or enjoy them lives in him, if he experiences anxiety, grief, anger or annoyance due to their absence or deprivation, then he is internally not free from them, and the fact that he possesses them, is contrary to the spirit of SADHANA.

Even being internally free from these things, he will not be ready to possess them, if he has not learned to use them not for himself, but for the sake of Divine Will - as a tool used through correct knowledge and action for the proper arrangement of a life that is not lived for himself. , but for the Divine and in the Divine.

Asceticism for the sake of asceticism is not the ideal of this Yoga, but self-control in the vital and proper order on the material plane are a very important part of it - and even ascetic discipline is more suited to our goal than licentiousness, a complete absence of true control.

Dominance over material goods does not mean that a person should generously scatter them or spoil them with full handfuls, as soon as they come to him or even faster. Dominance implies the correct and careful use of things, as well as self-control in their use.

If you want to practice Yoga, you must gradually take a yogic position in all matters, small and great. On our way, this position consists not in forceful suppression, but in disconnection from desire and impartiality, equal attitude towards its objects.

Forceful suppression (this includes limiting oneself in food) is a phenomenon of the same order as free connivance; in both cases desire remains: in one case it is fed by connivance, in the other it remains hidden and inflamed by suppression.

And only when you retreat from it, separate yourself from the lower vital, refusing to consider its desires and demands as your own, and also cultivate in relation to them a complete impartiality and equanimity of consciousness, the lower vital itself begins to gradually purify itself and become calm and impartial.

Each incoming wave of desire must be observed as quietly and with the same indestructible detachment, as if something was observed happening outside you - it must be allowed to pass, tear it away from consciousness and calmly put in its place true movement, true consciousness.

Attachment to food, greed for food and passionate craving for it, giving it excessive importance - this is what is contrary to the spirit of Yoga. There is nothing wrong with knowing that something tastes good; there should not be only desire or longing for it, exultation at its receipt, as well as displeasure or regret at its absence.

A person should be calm and impartial, not get upset or annoyed when the food is tasteless or not abundant - eating exactly as much as needed, no more and no less. There should be no craving or disgust.

Constantly thinking about food and keeping the mind occupied with it is a completely wrong way to get rid of the desire to eat. Give the food element the right place in life, a small corner, and do not focus on it, think about other things.

Don't preoccupy your mind with food. Take it in the right amount (not too much, not too little), without greed or disgust, as a means given to you by the Mother to maintain the body, and also with the right attitude, presenting it to the Divine in you; then she will not have to generate tamas.

The suppression of taste, rasa is by no means a part of this Yoga. What you have to get rid of is vital desire and attachment, greed for food, too much joy about getting food that you like, regret and discontent about not having it, giving food too much value. As in many other cases, impartiality is the criterion here.

The idea of refusing food that has visited you is a false inspiration. You can continue to get by with a small amount of food, but you cannot do without it at all, except for relatively short periods of time. Remember what the Gita says: "Yoga is not for the one who eats too much, and not for the one who refuses to eat at all."

Vital energy is one thing, it can be drawn in large quantities without food, and as a result of fasting it often increases; but the physical substance without which life loses its support is something else.

Do not ignore this side of nature (the desire to eat) and do not turn it into something special; it should be dealt with, cleansed and controlled, but not overly emphasized.

There are two ways to master it: the first is to practice disconnecting from desire, learning to view food as a purely physical necessity, and the vital satisfaction of the stomach and the taste of food as something insignificant; the second is the ability to take any food, without making preferences, and find in it (no matter how others say about it, good or bad) the same race - not the given food as such, but the universal Ananda.

It is a mistake to neglect the body by letting it gradually deteriorate; the body is an instrument of SADHANA and must be kept in good shape. We should not get attached to the material part of our

133

nature, but we should also not despise it or treat it with disdain.

The goal of this Yoga is not only union with the higher consciousness, but also the transformation (through its power) of the lower one, including the physical nature of man.

You don't need to have a desire or a strong craving to eat. The yogi does not eat under the influence of desire, but in order to maintain the body.

Indeed, in the presence of a strong mind and nerves or dynamic willpower with the help of fasting, one can temporarily enter a state of internal energy and receptivity that is tempting for the mind, but the usual reactions of hunger, weakness, intestinal disorders, etc. can be completely avoided.

But at the same time the body suffers from exhaustion, and an unhealthy state of overexertion can easily develop in the vital, due to an excessive influx of vital energy, which the nervous system is unable to assimilate or distribute. Nervous people should avoid the temptation of fasting, as they often experience hallucinations or loss of inner balance, or lead to them.

Fasting is especially dangerous if it is prompted by a feeling of protest or takes on the features of a hunger strike, for in this case it condones a vital movement that can easily become a bad habit detrimental to SADHANA. Even if these reactions were avoided, there is still not much benefit in fasting, since receptivity and energy from above should come through the tension of consciousness and a strong will for SADHANA, and not under the influence of artificial or physical means.

The transformation we are striving for is something too vast and complex to come at once; he needs to be given the opportunity to come in stages. Physical change is the last of these stages and, in turn, is a gradual process.

# Chapter 11: Yoga Meditation To Reduce Stress

Yoga meditation is a practice that involves calming and controlling your mind. It is a good way for you to be able to discover more about yourself and live a happy and peaceful life. The best thing about it is that it is not that hard to do, you just need to be able to concentrate better and make the most out of sitting still and not doing anything at all. If you are still not convinced about doing it, here are some of the benefits that you are going to get when you decide to try it.

Boosts your brain's power

One of the major benefits that you are going to get when you decide to practice meditation is that you are going to have a calm mind and you are going to be able to relax better. Meditation helps a lot when it comes to providing you with great experiences and feeling that gets sent to your brain so that you are going to be able to restore your energy and feel less stressed. A few minutes of meditation a day helps out a lot when it comes to improving your brain power and thus this is something that you really must check on and see how it is going to help you out.

Protects your brain

Another thing that you are going to get from it is brain protection which means to say that you are going to be able to keep away from all the cognitive disease and any mental decline that you might be experiencing. Regular meditation practice is surely going to be able to keep your mind on the right track so that you would not have to worry about dementia, Alzheimer's, and other diseases that might affect your memory.

Stimulates your brain

You are also going to help yourself out to be stronger, to be calmer and in the process, you are going to be more efficient at what you are going to do after it. Meditation is known to help the brain is being stimulated so that you are going to be able to learn more, have better memory, better compassion and increase your self-awareness and your introspect when it comes to a lot of things so this is a good thing to try out. This has been proven true by a lot of prestigious schools like Harvard so you might want to consider this.

Enhance concentration

In the case that you think you are having poor concentration skills; you might want to consider that meditation is known to be able to help you to improve it. It is going to enhance both your concentration and your attention so this will enable you to have a better quality of life. Surely, this is something that you want to consider as a great thing and reason to do meditation regularly as well.

After knowing more about the benefits that yoga meditation is going to be able to bring to you, the next chapter is going to give you a sample routine that you can try out to start your yoga journey.

# Chapter 12: Release Negative Or Stagnant Energy And Emotions

One of the beautiful gifts that yoga offers us is the opportunity to sit down with uncomfortable emotions and continue working with them. This is especially true for me when I develop a Yin yoga practice. Being trapped for 5-10 minutes not only releases the body physically, but we also find mental and emotional release. For people going through things from their past or current situations, this can be incredibly powerful and healing. It can also be excruciating to bring up these emotions, so I want to warn people to have other supports in creating space to allow painful feelings to arise.

In general, the following poses are great for helping you find a release, physical, mental, and emotional.

Hip openers

Vast numbers of us will, in general, store our feelings in the hip area. This is an essential piece of the "battle or flight" stress reaction. Every time we feel threatened or have a stress response, we respond physically by tensing ourselves in this area or pulling or fleeing to protect ourselves.

But even after the threat has passed, there is still an emotional scar from what triggered the situation. When we do not process these emotions, they remain stagnant and prevent us from moving forward.

The space between the hips is likewise the area of the second chakra or vitality focus. This chakra is connected to our associations with others, which are regularly the wellspring of troublesome feelings, be it deserting, hatred, or misfortune. At the point when the chakra is shut or uneven, you may see troubles in your connections and the sentiment of being trapped.Igniting this hip-opening chakra is a way to open yourself up to processing, find forgiveness, and understand the root of your emotions.

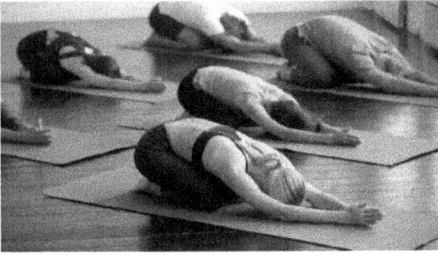

1. recline angle

You can rehearse this posture with or without embellishments. Having a pad under the spine makes it a heart opener just as a hip opener, which will expand the sentiment of discharge. I likewise prefer to rehearse this posture with one hand on my heart and the other on the space between my hips.

2. Pigeon pose

Pigeon is one of the most profound hip openers we practice in yoga, and regularly one of the most physical and mental difficulties. Utilize all the extras you need to feel bolstered and rest a little in the posture. Exploit that sentiment of help as a chance to celebrate and investigate unhesitatingly to let everything come to do that

.3. Child's attitude

Take this pose with your knees wide to create a hip opening. This posture is called so precise because it allows us to snuggle up and embrace a child's virtues. When we grow up, we allow ourselves to become vulnerable.

In this way, we can be used to it, without the need to impress, act, or react in any particular way. It is an invitation to withdraw to childhood and let our emotions flow freely as before.

Twists

Turns are convincing for processing and vigorously preparing things. As indicated by Ayurveda, the sister study of yoga, sound processing is fundamental; for the nourishment, we eat as well as for the encounters we gain.

These encounters can incorporate discussions with individuals, the earth around us, our reactions to things, all of which bring out our feelings. Rehearsing turns invigorates the stomach related framework and supports the activity of handling.

## 4. Turn supported

Use one large pillow or two smaller pillows and a blanket to create a beautiful, supportive bed. Bring one hip to the side of the pad and twist, bending your torso down. Bring both cheeks to the cushion. Focus on your breathing, and watch what happens. Actively relax all parts of the body and allow yourself to relax.

Relaxing poses where the body does not do much physically, except existing ones, are perhaps the most powerful. When the body is silent, the mind often wanders. Use this space to return thoughts to body and mind. Take an inventory of how the frame and state of mind feel.

If something becomes unbalanced, you start to become curious about why and what is the source of this feeling. Direct your attention to that discomfort and, instead of pushing it down, create the space to invite it.

## 5. Legs against the wall

This pose is such a sweet release; it purifies the energy in the body. We physically allow the legs to dissipate the old heat and mentally melt away the heaviness.

There are various varieties of this posture. You can begin altogether without frill, or attempt it with specific backings under the hips and the spine. You can likewise put a square on your feet for a little weight and a cover over your body for warmth and security.

6. Savasana

In such a rush in our lives to each other, we always do ourselves an invaluable favor when we can find complete silence. The mind needs these moments of silence to process and reflect. You have to remove the stimuli to understand all the things you need every day.

Instead of mentally spending your Savasana on your shopping list, try your best to be on your mind and body, it may be your only chance to do it all day. Silently watch what appears and be open to any significant changes that may occur.

Often we don't understand the cause of our emotions. We are not sure why we are angry, sad, or depressed. It may be that there is a profound and deep-rooted answer that we need time and space to understand. But making friends with your mind and body is one way to bring these things to the surface. Opening the parts of the body that contain these emotions is another piece of the puzzle. Try practicing these poses; They can lead you to a breakthrough that will give you some clarity and help you overcome your difficult emotions.

How to relieve aches and pains with yoga

Some of yoga's most obvious benefits include an incredibly taut body, more flexibility, and better balance. One of the other great benefits that are often overlooked is that it can also ease aches and pains.

Yoga can provide relief from a variety of different pains and conditions, including

Joint pain Headache Digestive problems Muscle pain or stiffness Back pain Knee pain Many other joint chronic pains

Keep in mind that improving flexibility is generally the best way to relieve most aches and pains, especially muscle aches and stiffness.

This requires repeated stretching of the muscles daily (best) or weekly (2-3 times per week). This helps to warm up the muscles and joints and reduce stress on the body.

Joint pain

Joint pain is probably the most common condition people face, and it mainly affects older or overweight people. It often stems from a variety of reasons, including a lack of essential nutrients, weak bones, and inadequate exercise. Some places where people often find pain are the knees, wrists, shoulders, and hips.

The knees and hips are the hardest hit because they are responsible for our balance and mobility.

Practicing yoga can help increase and strengthen the mobility and function of your joints. Some common yoga poses to practice include:

Triangular shapes

This stance is perfect for the entire body, as it reinforces the muscles around the knee, hip, and shoulder joints.

You can utilize a yoga obstruct for help on the off chance that you can't arrive at the ground serenely.

Ensure your back foot is forward and center around fixing your hips while gazing upward.

Hold for 10-20 seconds and rehash on the opposite side.

Warrior II works comparable muscles to Triangle yet additionally carries increasingly stretch to your quads.

Headache

Chronic headaches and migraines also plague many people, and this only gets worse as we continue to add more stress and distraction to our lives. Yoga has as many mental benefits as physical benefits. Meditation can do wonders to help you let go of life's many nuances and focus on the things that matter. A significant side effect of this is also the reduction of stress and anxiety.

Practice meditation regularly to ease some of these pains. If you find you need more, try the following:

Sitting forward bend

This posture can help ease some of the tension built up in your head and help you see again. It also works great to increase flexibility in your hamstrings!

Just focus on leaning forward as long as you can comfortably hold the pose, then hold it for 30 seconds. Repeat 3x for optimal effects.

If it is due to natural movements over time or previous injuries, knee movements come not only from the kneecaps and the surrounding muscles and joints but also from the quadriceps muscles.

Take care not to worsen knee pain. Make sure you enter the postures slowly and stop where you feel comfortable. If you feel more pain, ease the stretch.

Back pain

Back pain is the one I hear the most about grumblings, uncommonly low back torment. It torments such countless individuals and can be brought about by a wide range of components, for example, age, weight, and, most importantly, our chiefly inactive way of life. A great many people sit in the vehicle while in transit to work,, sit at a desk to work, sit during meals, and then come home and sit on the couch all night. Sitting can even cause strain on the neck and lower back. Compiled over time, it can cause chronic pain and other problems.

Cobra poses

This posture is delicate on the back, however but can also help strengthen it actively.

It is a pose with which you can choose to work or simply go through the movements actively. Be sure to stretch your back muscles consciously.

Lie on your stomach and place your hands on one foot in front of you, shoulder-width apart. Gently lift with core and back muscles.

# Chapter 13: Benefits Of Meditation

The practice of meditation originated in India between 5,000 and 3,000 BCE. Archeologists, while at the Indus valley, discovered evidence of meditation.

The images depicted people sitting in what could be recognized as meditation postures. They also discovered descriptions regarding meditation techniques that were found in the Indian scriptures that date back to 3,000 years ago.

Over the centuries the practice was adopted by some of India's neighboring countries where it formed part of the religions. It then spread to other parts of the region and is now practiced throughout the world.

While the practice of meditation varies depending on the cultural and religious influences, it has been identified as a significant cornerstone of spiritual development. The various aspects of meditation, including the mystical elements, has been incorporated by almost all the major religions.

One doesn't have to follow the religious traditions to enjoy the benefits of meditation, making it a universal act that can be practiced by anyone in the world.

The practice of meditation continues to rise in popularity due to numerous studies that have been conducted to reveal the various benefits.

Meditation should be practiced on a regular basis as a way to train the mind and improve concentration, focus, and to control your thoughts. Numerous benefits have been associated with the practice of meditation.

Along with clarity of mind, meditation can help improve your sleeping patterns, provide you with relief from depression, stress, and anxiety, enhance your levels of self-discipline, enhance your levels of positive mental attitude, as well as improve your mood.

There are many other valuable benefits that can be experienced through the practice of meditation. Just as in the same way that meditation alters the mind, it also changes the structure and functioning of the brain, resulting in various mental benefits.

There are numerous benefits of meditation, added to the fact that it can be done freely from the comfort of your own home, makes it extremely useful. Meditation provides spiritual, physical, mental, and emotional benefits. Here are some of the benefits you can gain from practicing meditation on a daily basis.

Mental Benefits

There are numerous mental benefits that are associated with regular meditation. Here are just a few of the mental benefits that you can gain by practicing mindfulness through meditation on a regular basis.

Reduces Stress, Anxiety, and Depression

One of the main reasons why people engage in meditation is to find relief from stress, depression, and anxiety. They have determined that meditation helps to reduce stress levels and depression, both mentally and physically.

When the body experiences a sudden threat or increased stress, it immediately triggers the fight or flight response. This leads to a sudden rush of adrenaline due to the release of epinephrine hormones.

These hormones cause your pulse rate and blood pressure to rise, and increases blood flow to your muscles, and results in faster breathing. The relaxation process that occurs during meditation helps relieve stress and the symptoms associated with stress.

After just eight weeks of consistent meditation practice, the benefits you gain are enormous and may even last for years.

Mindful meditation, when combined with breathing techniques has the potential for dramatically reducing or in some cases, eliminating cases of stress, anxiety, and depression that occur when the daily pressures of life and other unpleasant situations become greater than you can cope with.

Stress and depression don't occur because the situation at hand is valid or not. It is influenced more by how you respond to the situation. Practicing meditation gives you the opportunity to analyze the stressors and determine if they are valid or not.

Meditation creates a level of awareness where you are able to see things from another perspective. Training the mind through various meditation techniques will increase the mental resources that are used to help you in addressing stress and depression.

With consistent meditation practice, you can improve the clarity, focus, and calm in your mind, which leads to a reduction of stress. All that is required to be free from stress and depression is practicing meditation for about 10 minutes a day.

Recovery from Addiction

It has been proven that regular meditation practice can be extremely useful in helping with recovery from addiction. Meditation helps change how the brain is able to process information.

This helps to enable addicts to evaluate cases of addiction and allows them to act appropriately without the use of drugs. Mindful meditation helps to induce the state of relaxation, giving addicts the ability to monitor their breathing as they stay calm.

Being in this kind of state helps them to reduce negative feelings and the cravings that cause addicts to seek out the drugs or substances that they are addicted to. Anyone can learn the process of meditation for recovery from addiction.

Engaging in meditation helps those recovering from addiction to clearly observe their desires and thoughts without being compelled to act on them. It allows them to come to the understanding that they aren't responsible for the thoughts that come into their minds, but that they are responsible for how they ultimately react to those thoughts.

With the clarity of mind that meditation brings, addicts can make healthier choices that help in the recovery process.

During the early stages of the recovery process, addicts often experience severe mood swings. By engaging in meditation, their mind is forced to focus on one thing, such as breathing, a mantra, or an object that can help them to focus on overcoming addiction.

Reduces Pain

There have been various clinical settings that have used meditation to help patients that deal with chronic pain. Numerous studies have discovered that if you are capable of focusing and calming your mind and body that you are equally capable of controlling pain.

The practice of meditation makes it possible to face muscle tension, irritability, and sweating that is often associated with chronic pain. When you practice mindfulness through meditation, you are better able to come to terms with the pain that you are experiencing instead of running away from it or masking it with medication.

Increase Happiness

You can significantly increase your level of happiness and good feelings by engaging in mindfulness through meditation. Participating in regular practice will allow your brain to better focus on positive emotions.

Just like when you train your muscles and exercise for better performance, you can also work on your feelings of happiness. Engaging in meditation regularly increases your feelings of joy and happiness.

Mindful meditation helps to improve the psychological function of the brain, leading to the release of the hormones that are responsible for feelings of joy.

Health Benefits

The health benefits that are associated with meditation are pretty diverse. Some have even been proven scientifically to be extremely effective. Here are some of the health benefits that you can experience when you engage in meditation regularly.

Increased Immunity

It has been proven that when you get into a relaxed state through meditation, it helps to boost the immunity in patients that are recovering from cancer.

With the continued practice of muscular relaxation, you can reduce the risk of cancer coming back. It also helps to boost the natural killer cells that are common with the elderly, giving them a higher level of resistance to viruses.

Emotional Balance

Your emotional balance entails being free from the neurotic behavior that leads to a troubled ego. If you want to remain focused and find mental clarity, it is critical that you achieve emotional balance.

Meditation helps to cure cases of emotional imbalance, leading to the release of soaked memories, which then results in mental freedom.

Your reaction and responses to issues will no longer be influenced by the emotional burden when you start to practice meditation. It will allow you to view things in their true nature.

Lowers Blood Pressure

Practicing meditation has been shown to help with reducing blood pressure levels. It also helps to make the body become less responsive to the hormones that cause stress. Meditation provides similar results that can be experienced when taking blood pressure medication.

Engaging in meditation will help to significantly reduce stress levels, which enables your body's systems to normalize, resulting in overall improved health.

Improved Cardiovascular Health

When you are in a meditative, relaxed state, the release of nitric oxide by the brain increases. This causes the blood vessels to open up, resulting in a drop in blood pressure.

Nitric oxide is responsible for improving the function of the immune system, regulating blood pressure levels, improving the role of the central nervous system, behavioral activities, and improved memory.

Practicing meditation alters the physiological functioning of the body. This positively impacts some parts of the brain which results in experiencing deep levels of relaxation and calmness.

This deep level of relaxation results in the heart pumping blood slowly and steadily, delivering sufficient levels of oxygen throughout the body.

Spiritual Benefits

Many different religions have incorporated meditation into their religious practices. However, because meditation is more like a science, it can be practiced by anyone, regardless of their faith or religion.

There are numerous spiritual benefits that you can experience through the practice of meditation.

Increased Self-Awareness

One of the significant spiritual benefits of practicing meditation is self-awareness. Self-awareness involves going deep within yourself through mindful meditation, with the intention of connecting with your inner self.

Self-awareness forms the basis of meditation and entails being able to identify with the very core of being, being aware of the present moment, how you react to things, the subtle issues of the mind along with the behaviors and habits.

Once you are aware of this, you will learn how to keenly monitor how you respond to situations from a disconnected point of view.

Practicing meditation allows you to rise above the domain of your senses to connect deeper with the spirit.

Operating at this level supersedes the emotional level and provides you with the capability to usher yourself into a state of high revelation and insight, which isn't attainable at the emotional level.

# Chapter 14: The Healing Effects Of Sleep

Some believe the myth that we need less sleep as we age. We think sleeping three or four hours a night is enough to work correctly. If you wake up groggy or feel tired all day, you blame your busy lifestyle. They rely on caffeine to keep them alert and pledge to "catch up" during the weekend's sleep. The reality is that children, adolescents, and adults need more than a few hours of sleep each night. Chronic diseases, such as depression, hypertension, diabetes, and obesity, are more likely to occur in people who lack sleep. Indeed, rest is increasingly seen as critical to public health due to insufficient sleep concerning motor vehicle crashes, industrial incidents, and medical and other occupational mistakes.

The Importance of Sleep
 Like food and exercise, sleep is essential to optimal health and happiness. While

you rest, your brain stays active and is responsible for a wide range of biological maintenance tasks, which keeps your mind and body functioning and prepares you for the day ahead. The body needs time to heal, refresh, and detox properly. It is not enough time for your body to sleep just a few hours to get your body ready to work at its best. Some of the risks involved with inadequate sleep are as follows:

Short-term memory loss

Sleep privation will affect the memory for a short time and hurt your thought. You can forget about a task or stop halfway, forgetting what the original job was.

Depression

You may not be able to complete simple tasks if you lack motivation. The lack of energy and the loss of focus will contribute to a negative picture of yourself.

Weak Immune System

The sleep of the body is when tissues heal and rebuild, bone and muscle development, and the immune system is improved.

Metabolism and weight

Deprivation of chronic sleep can cause weight gain by disrupting the processing and storage of carbohydrates and altering hormone levels that influence our appetite.

Mood

Sleep loss can lead to irritability, impatience, lack of concentration, and mood. Too little sleep can also make you too exhausted to do stuff.

Cardiovascular Health

Hypertension elevated stress hormone levels, and irregular heartbeats have been associated with severe sleep disorders.

How much sleep is enough?

According to the National Sleep Foundation, although the needs for sleep differ a little from person to person, most healthy adults require between 7 and 9 hours of sleep per night to perform their best. The Foundation recommends that children in schools (5-10 years) require 10-11 hours of sleep every day, and teenagers (10-17 years) need 8.5-9.5 hours.

According to the National Health Interview results, almost 30% of adults reported an average of six hours or less per day of sleep. Just 31% of high school students reported sleeping for an average school night for at least 8 hours.

One of the biggest myths is that people can "take" sleep by sleeping during the weekend. It turns outweighs not that easy to recover from a chronic lack of sleep. It is not enough to get two good nights of sleep to pay off long-term debt. While extra sleep can be given a temporary boost, the day wears down your efficiency and strength.

How to get enough sleep hygiene

Tips For the sake of good sleeping habits and daily sleep,

"Sleep hygiene" is known. With this little effort and practice, the following tips on sleep hygiene will help you sleep well:

Go to bed every night simultaneously and get yourself up every morning. Coherence is critical. When you have a regular sleep schedule, you're much more rested and energized than sleeping at different times for the same number of hours.

Regular physical activity can contribute to sleep promotion, but a few hours before going to bed will be prevented.

Avoid big meals before going to bed.

Avoid close bedtime, caffeine, and alcohol. Evite nicotine.

Don't watch TV, cook, work, or use your room computers. Clear from the bedroom, all televisions, laptops, and other "gadgets."

Make sure the room is calm, dark, and soothing, not too hot or too cold.

If you're incredibly tired and can't function during the day, a short nap can help to relax and reset. Reduce your rest to thirty minutes as longer sleep can interfere with your sleep at night.

Try integrating the treatment of your mind and therapies like yoga, meditation, acupuncture, reiki, reflexology, and massage into your daily routine as well as having good sleep habits. Research has shown that these treatments relax the mind and ready the body for restorative sleep.

Relax with meditation and guided imagery

One thing that keeps people alert at night is that their mind is concerned. The brain releases the natural tranquilizing chemicals by using visualization for relaxation, and meditation, which renders directed imaging a usual way of reducing stress-related conditions, such as headaches, high blood pressure, pre-menstrual stress, and other stress-related psychological conditions.

Yoga

Research suggests that this ancient exercise can help fight against insomnia, reduce tension, and avoid aches and pains that can leave you tossing and turning all night long.

Reiki / Touch Healing Therapy

Reiki has based on Western philosophy that energy helps your natural healing ability. Reiki is a healing touch therapy. Reiki is a healing activity in which practitioners lightly or just above the individual to promote their healing response. Reiki sessions will help you relax and relax to prepare the way to better sleep.

Acupuncture

Acupuncture has a nervous system relaxing effect. It enhances sleep patterns by the clearing of muscle and nerve channel obstructions, encourages the release of oxygen-enriched energy, and relaxes the body.

Reflexology

operated by stress relaxation and suppressed energy release. The reflex point in the middle of the top pad in each broad toe refers to the pineal gland. A tiny cone-like organ that releases the hormone melatonin is the pineal gland. Since melatonin affects the sleep pattern of an individual, healthy sleep must maintain a balanced level.

Sleep - Why It Should Top Your Priority List

Most believe that rest is a waste of time. Nothing is going on, after all. All those hours in the night when you could do stuff! Here's why it's not only wrong; it's a risky line of thought.

It's not that nothing is going on during the night. A lot is going on! It's not that you go from the priority list of your body during exercise to no priority list during sleep. Alternatively, rest implies a change from the behaviors that reign during your day to the activities that rule during the night.

During sleep, the body allows all behaviors that do not occur in active mode "rest-and-digest" or "beat and raise." All those resources that were moved into operation are now allocated to these other roles during restful sleep. Are there any examples? The body builds bone in the night, rebuilding tissue, washing waste, combating bacteria, eliminating toxins, creating new cells.

When this turn isn't made in your automatic nervous system, you will eventually weaken and then burn out your pituitary gland, thyroid, adrenal glands, and gonads. This is achieved through two aspects of your automatic system that activate and inhibit those endocrine glands. It galvanizes the muscle system and the ability to react physically in the daytime or active mode. Their focus prioritizes cleaning and maintenance during the night or sleep mode.

Don't give this second agenda enough time, and you and your body are exhausted by the fact that different functions start to fail. As you start, do, do, fix, and repair your physical condition gets worse. This is the way it ends up in an early grave with a harrowing ride on the road.

The body requires much more extended periods of restorative-healing mode in cases, including childbirth, where the agency has a long list of recovery-repair work to do, including rehabilitation from emotional or physical shock or trauma.

During sleep, they are tasks that do not require quick responses, such as those controlled by your active-day (or sympathetic nervous system) agenda.

The rest healing (or parasympathetic mode) stimulates five body systems:

Lungs

Liver

Intestinal tract

Pancreas

Bronchial muscles
While, it inhibits these five glands:
The adrenal
Hypophysis
The nucleus
The thyroid
The ovaries
Why can't you sleep?
The common causes of the disease are:
Food allergies
Heavy metals
Petroleum solvencies
-Bacteria
-Viruses
-Yeasts
-Lyme vectors and cofactors
-Parasites
-Mold
Physical toxicity
EMF exposure (wireless internet links, mobile phones, smart meters, microwave stoves, etc.)
Medicines that activate your sympathetic system or inhibit your sympathetic system (the terms of online search indicate which ones).

Promoting restful sleep

Many necessary measures are available to support good night's sleep:

Avoid the main food intolerances; they are the lead producers of sympathetic superiority that is the different autonomic nervous mode to be used to cure sleep.

Do not eat stimulants in the middle of the afternoon. You can instead drink herbal teas soothing (chamomile or lemon bake are two examples of nerve soothing) or peppermint to improve your digestion.

Through your consumption of alkaline mineral products, as they help to slow down things, particularly if your body feels like racing.

Several sources are potassium, iodine, kelp, calcium, magnesium, and vitamin D. African berries, orange juice, bananas, dates, raisins, potatoes, and yams are a rich source of food.

Prevent overuse of sugar-for many reasons, this is always a good idea, but sugar is the primary cause of potassium depletion in terms of sleep.

Consider using diuretics and blood pressure drugs, as they also deplete potassium wherever possible.

# Chapter 15: Breathing Meditation

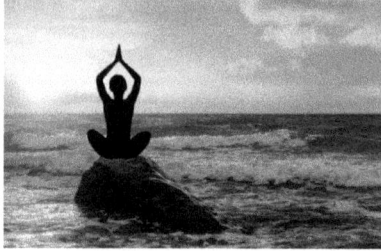

Breathing Meditation
When people think of meditation, they often think of nothing more than stopping one's thoughts. While not incorrect, meditation is so much more than this -- it can balance emotions, improve brain function, and allow the mind to be receptive to things beyond the normal spectrum of understanding. There is a lot of literature available on the topic of meditation, and unfortunately much of it is conflicting. People find a way that works for them and wrongly assume that it is the only way that it can be done, and this leads to confusion regarding technique

and method. In fact, finding what works for you is more important than doing it the way that anyone says you <sub>should</sub> be doing it. Meditation, in truth, is a form of brain training; and while there are many different ways to do it, one of the most common practices is something called Breathing Meditation.

The theory behind many forms of meditation is that by focusing all of your thoughts and energy on a single thing (known as 'one pointedness') you will effectively shut out all other sensation and still your mind. In the case of Breathing Meditation (also known as 'Mindful Breathing'), the thing focused on -- not surprisingly -- is one's own breath.

Historically the breath has been associated with the life force, and therefore the act of focusing on one's breath can be viewed more figuratively as focusing on one's very essence. As the act of breathing is a necessary and involuntary part of living, it is an ever-present cycle and as such very easy to focus on.

If you're thinking about attempting Breathing Meditation, a good place to start would simply be sitting in a comfortable yet firm position and keeping track of the number of seconds that you inhale and exhale (you could do this lying down, but it's best to sit up as you don't want to fall asleep while you are meditating).

You may either close your eyes or keep them partially open. If you keep them open be sure not to be looking at anything that may draw your mind away from your breathing. Count to ten in your mind, inhaling slowly but fully. Do the same as you exhale and you will have completed a single cycle of breath. Make sure to fill your lungs completely while inhaling and to empty them completely as you exhale. Your goal is to complete as many cycles of breath as you can without thinking of anything else. If you do have a thought, it is best to address it and let it pass, as attempting not to think of something often causes the mind to focus on it even harder.

It may take some time before you notice anything, but if you keep practicing you will begin to notice that you are able to complete more cycles of breath without a break in your concentration. You may also notice that you lose track of time, or possibly feel that you have lost time. This is due to your mind being stilled to the point that you enter a trance state. In a trance state you are somewhere between being awake and being asleep, but you are often completely unaware of your physical form and any outside stimuli.

A more advanced technique most often associated with Yoga is called Pranayama, the Sanskrit word for 'Control of Breath'. Pranayama requires you to alternate your breaths between nostrils, inhaling through one for a set number of seconds and exhaling through the other for a set number of seconds. The ratio varies, but a good starting place would be to inhale through your left nostril for five seconds while keeping your right nostril shut with your thumb, then exhale through your right nostril for five seconds while keeping your left nostril shut with your thumb.

Once you are able to do this for about fifteen minutes without any trouble, gradually increase the number of seconds for both inhale and exhale. Remember that your breath should always be slow and steady -- if you find yourself struggling, reduce the number of seconds!

If you are able to master basic Pranayama the next step would be to work on breath retention, or Kumbhaka. The principles of Pranayama remain the same, only now you are going to be retaining your breath between inhale and exhale. This is known as Antar Kumbhaka.

You can start by inhaling for five seconds, holding your breath for ten seconds, and then exhaling for five seconds. Like basic Pranayama, when you can do this for a length of time without struggling you may gradually increase the number of seconds for each step. Be very careful not to hold your breath for too long, as this can be very dangerous. If you begin to feel dizzy or experience pain or tightness in your chest, stop immediately.

The next step is to add a period of cessation after exhale, which is known as Bahya Kumbhaka. This is the hardest to master and also the most dangerous, as it requires you to force all of the air out of your lungs and then refrain from inhaling for a period of time. This can be done either with Pranayama alone or in conjunction with Antar. If you wish to practice Bahya by itself, simply complete a cycle of Pranayama, but instead of inhaling immediately upon exhaling you wait for several seconds before doing so. Though we began our practice of Antar with a duration of ten seconds, a five second period of Bahya is recommended until you are comfortable enough with the exercise to increase it. As with Antar, dizziness and pain or tightness in your chest are signs that you are extending Bahya for too long.

It is important to note that no form of Pranayama should be practiced without proper training first, as damage can be done to the lungs and going to long without oxygen can have a negative effect on your brain and other organs. That being said, there are many noted cases of Antar and Bahya being extended to the point of either a change in or loss of consciousness, but this must be strongly advised against due to possible ill effects on the body.

# Conclusion

Do you know you can consider practicing meditation techniques for weight loss before sticking to any new diet? This quick, cost-free approach will take tension and anxiety off your shoulders. Many people try to start anything to help their weight loss practice. Some of them just tend to lose weight quicker and cheaper. This is why weight loss meditation is such a smart practice. If you haven't talked about it, you might have to. Weight reduction meditation can be a safe and successful means of mindful eating and losing weight.

Guided meditation training can enable human beings to deal with stress and other unpleasant feelings, which in turn could contribute to a smoother and more calming healthier distribution of body fat. Of course, mindful meditation may not specifically decrease the abdominal fat, but by reducing the level of stress, the amount of cortisol, and other unhealthy habits, it works.

If you are thinking of trying meditation, then this book is for you as it has all the important information that you need to understand the meditation. This book will explain all steps that you need to take for starting this practice; for example, the first move is to pick a session than to choose the place or fix the timing, etc.

There are also various kinds of meditation, but all convey the same message and follow a simple method for calming the mind, taking time to relax, and becoming more mindful of your body at the present moment. To see which one fits well for you, you should try various approaches until you find the best meditation practice for you.

But keep in mind that no weight loss meditation exercise will help you lose weight without changes to your diet and lifestyle. The bottom line is mindful eating as you try to lose weight. A careful meditation program is sure to make the transition simpler and help you keep the weight down.

Meditation is something that everyone should use to improve their emotional and behavioral health. Without special facilities or memberships, you can do it everywhere. Alternatively, there are readily accessible meditation services and community groups that you can join to take benefit. There is also a wide range of models with varying strengths and advantages.

Trying out a meditation form that suits your time table is an ideal way to enhance your quality of life, even though you only have a few minutes per day to do so.